Parkinson Pete's Bookshelves

Parkinson Pete's Bookshelves

Reviews of Eighty-Nine Books about Parkinson's Disease

PETER G. BEIDLER

cp

coffeetownpress

Seattle, WA

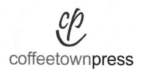

coffeetownpress

Coffeetown Press
PO Box 70515
Seattle, WA 98127

For more information go to: www.coffeetownpress.com

Cover design by Sabrina Sun

Parkinson Pete's Bookshelves
Copyright © 2018 by Peter G. Beidler—All rights reserved

ISBN: 978-1-60381-746-2 (Trade Paper)
ISBN: 978-1-60381-747-9 (eBook)

Library of Congress Control Number: 2017958900

Printed in the United States of America

for Marion Egge

for forty-five years

my student, friend,

co-laborer, collaborator

teacher

Contents

Shelf B: Nonfiction Books about Parkinson's by People with Parkinson's

Shelf C: Novels in Which at Least One Character Has Parkinson's

Preface: Sagging Bookshelves

I am by nature a reader of books. Not long after I was diagnosed with Parkinson's a dozen years ago, I began buying all the books about the disease that I could find. I soon noticed that they fell into three large categories of more or less equal numbers. I distributed the books among three shelves on my bookcase:

> Shelf A. Nonfiction books by people who do not have Parkinson's;
> Shelf B. Nonfiction books by people who have Parkinson's; and
> Shelf C. Fiction (novels) in which at least one character has Parkinson's.

I found some overlap in the books on Shelves A and B. Where should I put a book that was written by a medical doctor who was eventually diagnosed with Parkinson's? What about a book with multiple authors, one of whom had Parkinson's? In the end, I put such books on Shelf A if they emphasized the scientific and technical aspects of the disease. I put them on Shelf B if they emphasized the more personal aspects.

At the beginning I found myself wanting to read especially the books on Shelf A. I wanted facts, information about my disease and its history, about the medicines I might take, the surgeries I might be eligible for, the long-term prognosis, the likelihood of a cure. As I read the books on Shelf A, however, I sometimes found myself feeling like I was all body, no spirit. I sometimes felt that I was being talked down to by people who sometimes seemed to be more interested in my disease than in me. After that, I found myself drawn to the books on Shelf B, books written by people with my disease. I wanted to hear from people like me who knew what it felt like to have Parkinson's, who had experienced first-hand the confusion and the terror that comes with the diagnosis. I wanted not so much scientific facts by supposedly dispassionate doctors and other professionals, but information and advice from other people who had walked in my trembling footsteps and stumbling shoes. And then I found myself picking up the novels on Shelf C. These were books that told a story, often an exciting story, about people who had Parkinson's. I found that the Shelf C books were particularly useful in portraying two kinds of nasty reality that the writers of both Shelf A and Shelf B tended to shy away from. One of these was the stresses that Parkinson's visits on families of men and women with Parkinson's. The other was how people in the later stages of the disease live and how they die.

I had a lot of books on my sagging shelves, but I had no way of knowing which books were most useful or most reliable. I found no central location that guided me to read one book rather than another, that gave me information about the contents and presumed audience for each book, that gave me a thumbnail assessment of the various books on my three Parkinson's bookshelves. In the end, I decided that the thing for me to do was to read all of the books and make my own assessments. While I was at it, I decided to write short reviews of each of them. Partway through I offered a few of my reviews to the Northwest Parkinson's Foundation in Seattle for publication on their website or in their newsletter.

The encouraging comments that I received suggested to me that my collected reviews might be of use to others who have Parkinson's, to members of their families, to their friends, to their employers—to anyone who wanted to find out more about the disease. Reference librarians might appreciate having access to my collected reviews so they could direct their patrons to an independent description and assessment of the books. And doctors might like to have at hand a compendium like mine so they could tell their newly-diagnosed patients and their families—still in shock about the frightening new diagnosis—that there were not only a lot of books out there but also an informational guide to what those various books contained.

All but three or four of the reviews that I publish here appear in print for the first time. To give readers a sense of the style and approach of the various authors, I quote generously from most of the books. I have made no attempt to rank-order the books. Such a ranking would be arbitrary and would take no account of the fact that we all need to consult different kinds of books at different stages of the disease. The point is not to impose on others my quirky likes and dislikes, but rather to help readers choose which ones are most likely to give them the information they seek. If my evaluation is important to you, you will probably be able to tell from the tone of my reviews which ones I was most impressed with and which ones I was most skeptical about.

I list the books chronologically—from oldest to most recent—on each of the three shelves. Most of the books appeared in the twenty-first century, though for each of the three shelves I list one older book. If more than one book was published in a given year, I list them alphabetically by title in that year. Most of the ellipses indicate words that I left out and are enclosed in square brackets, as […] here. Where the ellipses are in the original, I omit the brackets, as … here. Like most writers, I prefer the term "Parkinson's disease" to the term "Parkinson disease." I use the latter only when I quote someone who uses it. Similarly, I use the terms "Parkie" and "PWP" (person with Parkinson's) only when I quote someone who uses those terms. Some writers capitalize terms like Qigong and some don't. I tend in my reviews to follow the practice of the writer of the book I am reviewing. I generally use the title "Dr." only for people who have a medical degree.

Shelf A: Nonfiction Books by People Without Parkinson's

A1. *Parkinson's Disease: The Complete Guide for Patients and Caregivers*, **by Abraham N. Lieberman, MD, Frank L. Williams, Susan Imke, Ellen Moscinski, Paula Benoist Falwell, Harley Gordon, with Suzanne LeVert. Fireside Book (Simon and Schuster), 1993. 270 pp.**

> "With a little luck and a lot of diligence, one of these futuristic procedures may end up proving to be a cure for Parkinson's disease, perhaps even within your lifetime."

How do eight people write a book together? If they do, whose name gets listed first and whose last? The answers to such questions can vary from book to book and from publisher to publisher, but for this book and this publisher the person whose name is listed first is the one with the medical degree—that would be Dr. Abraham N. Lieberman—while the person whose name is listed last is the one who did the actual writing—a professional health-topics writer named Suzanne LeVert. Apparently she consulted with the other seven as needed for certain topics and for checking drafts of her chapters as she wrote them.

In a twenty-five-year-old book of less than 300 pages with the title *Parkinson's Disease: The Complete Guide for Patients and Caregivers*, we neither expect nor get "completeness" in any meaningful sense of the term.

To say that is not necessarily to be critical of the book. Sometimes we want to skim the surfaces and get a broad overview of a subject.

Parkinson's Disease contains ten chapters. In the first three chapters we find a basic introduction to the disease: its history, its causes, its symptoms, its progression through various stages. The next two chapters discuss various ways to improve life for people with the disease—drugs, diet, exercise. The sixth chapter deals with the emotional adjustments that come with a diagnosis of Parkinson's: the panic, the sense of unfairness ("Why me?"), the gradual acceptance, the decisions about who to tell about your diagnosis and when to tell them, the benefits of a support group.

Most useful for most readers will be Chapter 7, a sixty-page chapter alphabetically listing almost every imaginable symptom and side effect, from "Aches and Pains," "Bathing and Bathroom Organization," "Bed Mobility," and "Constipation" (120–24) to "Vision Problems," "Writing," and "Zest and Zeal" (175–76). Here, by way of example, is the full entry on "Driving":

> If you were a good driver before your diagnosis, you're likely to remain a good driver for years to come, unless your disease progresses quite rapidly. Unfortunately, your limited mobility may diminish your driving skills at some point. Moving your foot back and forth from the brake pedal to the gas pedal may be slowed considerably. You may not be able to turn your head from side to side quickly or look out the back windshield. In addition, the medications you take to alleviate PD symptoms may make you sleepy from time to time, which certainly affects your driving skills. Once your reaction time and line of vision are so hampered, driving becomes hazardous. If you have any questions about your driving ability, attend a driving school to have your skills assessed by professionals.
>
> Giving up your driving privileges may be very difficult for you, since it will diminish your independence to some degree. Remember though, that nothing is more important than your safety and the safety of others. If you do give up driving, you'll soon find many other transportation options: public buses or subways, taxicabs, willing friends and relatives. Accept these options cheerfully and use them often; do not let your inability to drive isolate you from your favorite activities. (133)

That is all good advice, of course, but how many of us need to be given such advice? Is there anything in those two paragraphs that we did not already know?

The last three chapters present advice about the welfare of caregivers, about taking stock of your financial future in view of the upcoming and ongoing medical expenses you will encounter, and research and surgical activities that show at least some possible promise of leading to a cure for Parkinson's. It is but a slender promise, however, and Suzanne LeVert was wise not to overstate it: "With a little luck and a lot of diligence, one of these futuristic procedures may end up proving to be a cure for Parkinson's disease, perhaps even within your lifetime" (228). That was written twenty-five years ago. Most of the first audiences for *Parkinson's Disease: The Complete Guide for Patients and Caregivers*, if they are still alive, know that neither luck nor diligence have given them a cure. Newly-diagnosed patients today will find some general help in this book, but they will know better than to place too much hope in vague predictions about a cure in their own lifetime.

A2. *Parkinson's Disease and the Art of Moving*, by John Argue. Oakland, California: New Harbinger Publications, 2000. ix + 220 pp.

> "Through actions and exercises that you will do with your body, you will actually be training your mind."

If there is one therapy for Parkinson's disease that everyone agrees about it is that people with Parkinson's should exercise. Move. Walk. Go to the gym, Bike. Dance. Pump iron. Box. Do yoga. Do Tai Chi. As my friend Terry puts it, "We need to take the park out of Parkinson's." I don't know of a single neurologist who advises sitting around when we could be walking around.

Marion Jackson Brucker, a Parkinson's patient in Berkeley, helped to start a new kind of Parkinson's support group. She describes her experience in "Marion's Story: A Personal Experience with Parkinson's Disease," which serves as a kind of foreword to John Argue's *Parkinson's Disease and the Art of Moving*. She describes her own early experience with Parkinson's and with a disappointing neurologist who was interested only in treating her motor symptoms, not in her ideas or her aspirations to play the piano. Especially interesting is what Marion Jackson Brucker says about seeing Parkinson's as a progressive erosion of the body's ability to move automatically. Whereas we used to be able to walk down the sidewalk as we talked to a companion or sang a song or thought about a book we were writing or chewed bubble gum, we now needed to focus on just the walking. We had to consciously tell our left foot to go here, then tell the right foot to go there. If we took our attention away from the left-foot-right-foot movement to tell our walking companion that it might rain, or to wonder if that cat up ahead was a good mouser, or figure out where to spit out our bubble gum, our feet tended to freeze and we fell down. To continue to move effectively, we had to—by the power of the will—get our bodies to do what they had once done automatically.

Marion Jackson Brucker found a more compatible neurologist who listened to her ideas about a new kind of support group:

> A support group could be more than just a discussion group. What I needed was a support group with lessons in conscious movement and voice that would allow me to work within my limitations (Parkinson's disease) while at the same time encouraging me to wring the most out of what I could still do. Such a support group could be like so many art classes I had taken: it could be a structured series of classes that would teach people conscious ways to move and speak. We would be learning a kind of art form—something like acting maybe, with singing and yoga and dance and other things I hadn't thought of yet—to function better within our PD-imposed limitations. (8)

The new neurologist encouraged her. The man she tapped to guide her and eventually to run her support group was not a medical man or a physical therapist, but an actor, a theater man, a teacher named John Argue.

John Argue eventually wrote his ideas down, added photographs of himself doing the various poses and exercises, and published these in *Parkinson's Disease and the Art of Moving*. His title is carefully chosen. It is not *Exercise as Therapy for People with Parkinson's Disease* or *Move or You'll Die*. He wants us to view moving as an art form, an expression of our essential creativity: "In order to deal with your Parkinson's related difficulties, which derive from the loss of automatic movements, you need to learn to move and speak *consciously*" (15). He wants us to think of movement not as something that is good for the body but as something that is good for the mind:

Calisthenics, aerobics, and weightlifting are all important exercises if you wish to lose weight, put on muscle, keep in shape, or build stamina. Those are all legitimate goals, but they are not focused on your Parkinson's problem. The goal of this program is different: you are aiming at developing a mental ability. Through actions and exercises that you will do with your body, you will actually be training *your mind*. [...] Your overall goal—your strategy for coping with whatever symptoms come along—will be to develop an *artful* way of moving and speaking. An artful action is one that is *graceful, mindful, and complete*. (16–17)

The bulk of *Parkinson's Disease and the Art of Moving* is taken up with ten chapters or "lessons" (175 pages), each dealing with a different set of activities:

1. Sitting Exercises (The Warm-up)
2. Voice and Speech (The Cooldown)
3. Floor Exercises
4. On Hands and Knees
5. Leg Stretches
6. Going to the Floor
7. Standing Steady
8. Power Stances
9. Balance and Recovery
10. Walking, Freezing, and Turning

I am guessing that in John Argue's own classes his movement routines work amazingly well. He sounds like an accomplished, dramatic, charismatic, and inspirational teacher. I doubt, however, that his movement routines will work nearly as well for those working alone with just his book to guide them, or in a class run by someone else. There is a 189-minute color video available for those who want to order it and use it at home, but it would not be the same.

In the short appendix to his long book, John Argue writes:

At the first meeting of a new class, some student will inevitably ask, "Do you have Parkinson's?" to which I reply, "No, but I have several other things wrong with me!" (217)

I am troubled by that reply. It seems to assume as a given that to have

Parkinson's is to have "something wrong" with one. And it seems to assume further that for a teacher to guide people with Parkinson's effectively, he or she must also have "something wrong." That seems to me an unnecessarily negative way of thinking about having Parkinson's and about having the qualifications to teach people who have Parkinson's. I would have preferred a more positive reply, something like, "No, I don't have Parkinson's, but I have learned a lot about Parkinson's by working with people who do have it, and I never cease to be bowled over by the amazing strides people with Parkinson's can make with a little hard work and encouragement. So, let's get started!"

A3. *Parkinson's Disease: A Guide for Patient and Family* (fifth edition), by Roger C. Duvoisin, MD, and Jacob Sage, MD. Philadelphia: Lippincott Williams & Wilkins, 2001. ix + 182 pp.

> "The implications are profound. The most important is that for the first time in history we hold the keys that can unlock the mysteries of the basic mechanisms underlying this and related inherited diseases and thereby find methods of arresting, preventing, and even curing them."

There are lots of books about Parkinson's disease. Many of them cover the same general body of information: what is Parkinson's, what do we know about the causes of the disease, how does the disease typically progress, what medications and surgeries are available, how important is exercise, how can patients avoid being depressed as the disease progresses, what is the outlook for a cure? No two books have quite the same approach or make quite the same kind of contribution. *Parkinson's Disease: A Guide for Patient and Family* will be of value particularly for readers who are interested in two kinds of information about the disease: (1) the history of the disease and of the various approaches to it, and (2) the extent to which Parkinson's is a genetic disease.

The first edition of *Parkinson's Disease: A Guide for Patient and Family*, was published 1n 1978—almost four decades ago. It was written by Dr. Duvoisin. Dr. Sage was not taken on as co-author until the fourth edition in 1995. The field has changed dramatically since 1978, and even the most recent edition, the fifth, is now fifteen years old. Partly because of the long publishing history of the book, the authors have witnessed some of the major changes in the field, such as the emergence of carbidopa/levodopa, what is often called now the "gold standard" medication for Parkinson's, and the development of deep brain stimulation (DBS). The book gives its readers an unusually good historical sense of the disease.

Duvoisin and Sage, both of whom are or have been affiliated with the Robert Wood Johnson Medical School in New Brunswick, New Jersey, take us back two hundred years to James Parkinson's original 1817 article on the disease. Parkinson called it "the shaking palsy," but later physicians renamed it Parkinson's disease in his honor. The disease now includes a constellation of variously distributed symptoms like tremor, stiffness, slowness, leaning forward and other postural irregularities, imperfect balance and strange gait patterns, handwriting and vision problems, urinary, sexual, and digestive problems, problems with voice, drooling, and swallowing, freezing, stumbling, falling, and various mood and memory issues. Most of us have heard the term "Lewy body," but this book helpfully tells us that they are called that because in 1908 a man named Dr. Frederick Lewy noticed an aberration in certain degenerated nerve cells in the autopsied brains of people who shared certain symptoms of dementia. Duvoisin and Sage also tell us about the various medicines and procedures used before the discovery of levodopa in the 1960s.

The chapter on surgical treatments of Parkinson's gives a fascinating but rather frightening history of various efforts—mostly unsuccessful—to operate on the brain. Some of the early operations did seem, for a time, to relieve tremors and rigidity, but did so only temporarily and sometimes with disastrous side effects. As the authors put it:

> Many thoughtful physicians were disturbed by the idea of injuring the brain and causing further change in function, which was also poorly understood. Brain surgery could not cure or even alter the further progress of Parkinson's disease, and it relieved only some symptoms, mainly tremor and rigidity. Moreover, the operation had to be done twice, once for each side, if the symptoms on both sides were to be relieved, and complications were much more frequent when both sides were operated on. (109)

The authors tend to be cautiously conservative in their warnings about the dangers of brain surgery: "Surgery should be considered only after

all reasonable medical options have been tried and proved inadequate
to control the symptoms and complications of Parkinson's disease. The
complications of surgery can be devastating, including stroke, bleeding
in the brain, seizures, confusion, speech abnormalities, worsening of the
target symptoms, and even death" (112). DBS technology has advanced
considerably since 2001, but of course it is still wise to be cautious when
contemplating brain surgery.

Historians tend to look back so that they can look ahead. One of the
most fascinating chapters in *Parkinson's Disease: A Guide for Patient and
Family* is Chapter 14, "A Historical Perspective." This chapter traces the
various accidental and on-purpose discoveries in the past two centuries
that have led to the current understanding of Parkinson's. Of particular
interest is the account of the strange doings of a young narcotics addict
in Arlington, Virginia. An amateur chemist, he one day concocted out of
simple chemicals in his home lab a brew that he then self-administered.
The mixture caused him to become rigid and immobile. He was admitted
to a local hospital. The physician on duty, thinking that the young man's
symptoms resembled those of a person with Parkinson's, prescribed
carbidopa/levodopa. It worked—sort of. Subsequent investigation into the
concoction the young man had made and taken led to certain discoveries
about a by-product called MPTP. Though the young man died a year later
from a drug overdose, a post-mortem examination of his brain showed that
certain nerve cells deep in his brain had been wiped out.

A few years later, several drug addicts in California showed up in an
emergency room with what seemed to be sudden-onset parkinsonism. An
analysis of the drug they had taken showed that it also contained MPTP.
Researchers hoping to discover what caused Parkinson's conducted a
number of studies involving MPTP. They were not successful in isolating
through their MPTP research the exact cause of the disease, and thus were
not successful in finding a cure. But in a roundabout way their research
began to point in another direction: the possibility that there might be a
stronger genetic cause of the disease than had previously been supposed.

In Chapter 15, "Genetics: A Family Condition?" Duvoisin and Sage
discuss the implications of the fact that about a quarter to a half of the
people who have Parkinson's have at least one other close family member—
parent, a sibling, an aunt or uncle—who also had the disease. The chapter
opens with this arresting paragraph:

> That the cause of Parkinson's disease may lie within ourselves
> and be part our genetic inheritance transmitted to us down the

millennia through countless generations is an awesome thought
to contemplate. The very idea that it may be due to a minor defect
in our DNA, an error in our genetic code, that may be even more
ancient than our own species Homo sapiens, strikes at the very
depth of our sense of being. It may take time and patience to come
to terms with so breath-taking an idea, but as a result of advances
in the genetics of Parkinson's disease achieved in the last decade,
it has become clear that genes play a major role in its cause. The
implications are profound. The most important is that for the first
time in history we hold the keys that can unlock the mysteries of the
basic mechanisms underlying this and related inherited diseases and
thereby find methods of arresting, preventing, and even curing them.
(152)

In studies of large families with several individuals who had
Parkinson's, researchers have discovered some suspicious gene mutations,
but these do not occur frequently enough to serve as pathways to a cure.
Researchers have, however, discovered a mutation in the alpha-synuclein
protein that appears in the DNA of most people with Parkinson's. That fact
may someday contribute to a cure, but for now we are left with a series
of questions. If one person in a family has Parkinson's, how likely is it
that someone else in the family will have it or get it? (About fifty-fifty.)
Should others in that family be warned, watched, or tested for the disease?
(Probably not, since there is no reliable pre-symptomatic test and no cure
even if there was one.) Should a parent with the disease refrain from having
children because of the possibility that a child will one day develop full-
blown Parkinson's? (Don't be silly!)

A4. *Shaking Up Parkinson Disease: Fighting Like a Tiger, Thinking Like a Fox,* **by Abraham N. Lieberman, MD. Boston: Jones and Bartlett Publishers, 2002. xiii + 250 pp.**

> "Picture being in a car and the car won't start when you turn the key. Or, after it starts, the brake, not the accelerator, kicks in. You can't leave the car—because the car is you."

Dr. Abraham Lieberman had polio when he was six years old and subsequently spent eighteen months in various hospitals, rehab centers, and clinics. He eventually went to medical school, taught at New York University and the University of Miami. Dr. Lieberman became especially interested in Parkinson's disease and became medical director of the National Parkinson Foundation. He also helped set up and manage the Muhammed Ali Parkinson Research Center in Phoenix. As he puts it in his preface, because of his early experience with polio, he "knows adversity, anxiety, depression, fear, panic, and hope as a neurologist and as a patient" (x).

Shaking Up Parkinson Disease has a good bit of useful information about Parkinson's. Dr. Lieberman defines the disease in the standard way by listing the four most common characteristics of Parkinson's: tremor, rigidity, slowness, and postural instability. He describes some of the secondary symptoms, like difficulty in walking (irregular arm swing, stooped posture), problems with voice (softness, articulation), and with handwriting (tiny words, illegibility). He seems to get sidetracked from time to time, as when he wonders why so many famous people get Parkinson's, whether Adolf Hitler had the disease, and the validity of the so-called five "stages" of the disease.

Dr. Lieberman seems to want to discuss in puzzling detail a number of issues that most neurologists spend little or no time talking about: the lungs and shortness of breath (pages 55–60), drooling and swallowing (pages 60–70), constipation and bladder difficulties (pages 71–78), and sexuality (pages 78–84).

In the section on sexuality, for example, Dr. Lieberman talks about the "four phases of the human sexual response: 1) Excitement or arousal, 2) Plateau, 3) Orgasm, 4) Resolution" (78). He has sections on "Age, Sex, and Parkinson"; "Do Not Let Parkinson Kill Romance"; "Folk Remedies to

Put You in the Mood"; "Can Hormones Put You in the Mood?"; "Are Bad Arteries Keeping You From Being Aroused?'; "Are Drugs Keeping You From Being Aroused?"; "Arousal and the Autonomous Nervous System"; "So Why Can't I Become Aroused?"; and "Impotence." Under this last, he has four subheads: "How Common Is Impotence in Parkinson Disease?"; "Is It Parkinson or Something Else?"; "How Do I Tell My Doctor I'm Impotent?"; and "Viagra."

In Chapter 5 Dr. Lieberman distinguishes Parkinson's disease from disorders it is sometimes confused with: essential tremor, multiple systems atrophy, progressive supranuclear palsy, eye problems, restless legs, various kinds of dystonia.

In Chapter 6 he talks about what little is known about what causes Parkinson's. He notes that the five states with the highest per capita incidence of Parkinson's—North and South Dakota, Nebraska, Iowa, and Minnesota—are heavily agricultural states that use lots of chemical fertilizers, pesticides, and herbicides. He notes that there is a strong link between Vietnam veterans who had contact with Agent Orange and those who developed Parkinson's. By way of explaining why more men than women get Parkinson's, Dr. Lieberman discusses a possible link between estrogen and Parkinson's. He ends the chapter on causes with this thought: "Why do so many things cause Parkinson? To what end? To what good? In time we will know—and benefit" (131).

In the last three chapters—7, 8, and 9—of *Shaking Up Parkinson Disease*, Dr. Lieberman discusses three topics that he feels particularly strongly about: anxiety, depression, and dementia. Because these three chapters take up almost half of the pages in his book. they merit particular mention. First, he sees a strong connection between anxiety and Parkinson's: "Anxiety aggravates PD through the autonomous nervous system. During times of anger, fear, rage or stress when the heart beats faster, blood pressure rises, hands shake more than usual, and the patient feels they are about to die—it is not PD; it is the autonomous nervous system, and it can be treated" (133). Second, Dr. Lieberman sees a strong connection between Parkinson's and depression. Like anxiety, he says, depression can be treated: "Many of the ways of reducing anxiety can reduce depression. If you are depressed, meditation, counseling, exercise, and breathing techniques [...] may help you" (172). Third, Dr. Lieberman sees a strong connection between Parkinson's and dementia: "The outward features of dementia are obvious: confusion, memory loss, unusual behavior, and daytime drowsiness. [...] The economic cost of caring for a PD person with dementia is ten times the cost of caring for a PD person without dementia. The emotional and spiritual cost of caring for a PD person with dementia cannot be measured" (187). Dr. Lieberman points out that "Until recently, dementia has been an unspoken secret of PD. The attitude was, 'Why tell a person who's been diagnosed with PD he's at risk for dementia? At present there's no treatment for dementia'." He offers only the most unconvincing reason for hope: "At present, there is no drug that will delay the dementia of PD. But if history's a guide, in the next few years, such drugs will become available" (197). That was 2002.

Much of *Shaking Up Parkinson's Disease* is technical and beyond the comprehension of many of the readers the book was apparently intended for: "the puzzled, the hopeful, the willing, and the prepared" (i). There are, however moments of refreshingly lucid writing, as in the preface, where Dr. Lieberman uses a metaphor to describe what it is like to have Parkinson's: "Picture being in a car and the car won't start when you turn the key. Or, after it starts, the brake, not the accelerator, kicks in. You can't leave the car—because the car is you. And if someone, a doctor, jump-starts you with a drug, you'll do well—for a while—and then you're stuck again. [...] and you pray—yes you pray. For as important as science is, belief is equally important" (iii).

I close this review with reference to Dr. Lieberman's oft-repeated assertions of the importance of the Bible (see, for example, pages 7, 12, 33, 99). "People ask, if God created the world, and if God is good, why did God create Parkinson disease? [...] Read Isaiah; God has a purpose, we may not understand it" (110). "Why do so many things cause Parkinson? To what end? To what good? In time we will know—and benefit. Isaiah wrote: *"Who measured the water of the sea in the hollow of His Hand?"* [...] *"Who but God?"* (131); "When facing a disease like Parkinson, where anxiety increases and sleep is disrupted, do not forget the Bible. With the Bible's help and the help of science you will reach the state of what Isaiah dreamed: *When the eyes of the blind shall be opened, / And the ears of the deaf unstopped"* (153); "If you are a caregiver, and caregiving is difficult, look to God. Read the Bible. The Bible [...] is, like life, a repository of wisdom. Anyone can believe when things go well. But when things go badly, it is even more important to believe" (185); "In this, a dark hour, do not forget the Bible, or God. Listen to Jeremiah: [...] *"For I am God, who acts with faithful love"* (213).

It seems strangely out of place in a book about Parkinson's for a medical doctor to insist upon the importance of reading the Old Testament. Did he assume that Muslims, Christians, Hindus, Buddhists, and atheists who have Parkinson's are beyond help?

A5. *What Your Doctor May Not Tell You about Parkinson's Disease: A Holistic Program for Optimal Wellness*, **by Jill Marjama-Lyons, MD, and Mary J. Shomon. New York: Warner Books, 2003. xxvii + 414 pp.**

> "In contrast, complementary medicine looks at the causes and the nutritional and environmental factors that may aggravate or trigger disease in general and Parkinson's in particular."

There is much that is good and useful in *What Your Doctor May Not Tell You* about Parkinson's Disease, but I am troubled by the ambiguity of "may not tell you." Does it mean that your doctor *is not permitted to* tell you certain things about Parkinson's, or that your doctor *may be withholding* from you certain things about Parkinson's? I am troubled by the implication that you should distrust your doctor as being either ignorant or deceptive and that if you read this book you will learn certain secrets that will keep you healthy.

What is most distinctive in Dr. Jill Marjama-Lyons's book is her insistence on moving beyond the traditional Western approach to Parkinson's, an approach that treats it as primarily a physical disorder: "So much of the emphasis on treating a person with Parkinson's disease is on the physical symptoms—the tremor, muscle slowness, and rigidity—and little, if any, emphasis is put on the emotional, mental, and spiritual health of the patient" (xxii). That said, Dr. Jill, as she calls herself, spends most of her long book explaining the Western approach to the disease.

Much of that explanation is pretty technical. In Chapter 1, pages 5–10, for example, she refers to "substantia nigra compacta," "oxidative stress," "antioxidants," "free radicals," "mitochondria," "glutathione," "peroxides," "alpha-synuclein," "ubiquitin ligase," "excitotoxicity," and "apoptosis." She serves up these two sentences: "Specifically, MPP+ inhibits NADH (nicotinamide adenine dinucleotide hydrogen), which blocks the formation of ATP (adenosine triphosphate), the key energy molecule of all cells" and "The medications used to treat Parkinson's disease may be dopamine (carbidopa/levodopa is a precursor to dopamine, meaning it is converted by enzymes into dopamine), look like dopamine (dopamine agonists), or act on the enzymes that metabolize dopamine (MAO and COMT inhibitors)." Perhaps Dr. Jill felt that she needed to establish her credentials as a Western-style physician by using such terminology so early in her book, before moving on to what interested her most, alternative and complementary therapies.

Actually, I found Dr. Jill's explanations of the various Parkinson's symptoms and Western medicines to be generally comprehensive, usually clear enough, and quite helpful. It is obvious that she has no desire to replace conventional Western chemical and surgical treatments for Parkinson's, but seeks rather to augment them with other more "holistic" or "integrative" approaches:

> The basic idea is to view the person and his or her condition as all part of a whole, a system. This differs from the conventional Western medicine approach which is to focus solely on the disease and focus all treatment specifically on the disease. [...] In contrast, complementary medicine looks at the causes and the nutritional and environmental factors that may aggravate or trigger disease in general and Parkinson's in particular. (156)

Dr. Jill speaks of Chinese traditional medicine, including acupuncture and tai chi. She speaks of traditional Indian approaches, sometimes called ayurvedic medicine, including meditation and yoga. She speaks of herbal medicines and homeopathic and naturopathic approaches. She speaks of dietary, nutritional, vitamin, enzyme, and hormone therapies. She speaks of physical therapy, massage, and, of course, exercise.

In this short review I cannot attempt to give extended discussions of any of these, but I will say that Dr. Jill makes a strong case for trying some approaches, not as replacement for Western-style chemical and surgical options, but as complementary ones. And she makes a convincing case for the importance of a positive emotional and spiritual outlook in dealing with Parkinson's. I confess, though, that I was vaguely troubled by some of what she says about the role of spirituality.

In her introduction Dr. Jill says, "before I began writing this book, I meditated and I prayed for guidance. I wanted this book to be helpful to those who read it, something that would hopefully make a positive difference, even if in a small way. And the message I received was very clear—spirituality had to penetrate and permeate this book. It had to be found in every chapter, on every page, in every word" (xxii). In fact, however, she says little about spirituality until her last chapter, which she calls the "Epilogue." "We are all spiritual beings," she says, "and as such we all have a connection to one another, to God—whether you view God religiously or more in the sense of universal energy or life force—and all living things" (329). She says that "the power of faith, prayer, love, and hope is immeasurable. In fact, Western medicine is just now starting to catch up with this idea" (330).

Dr. Jill quotes Faye, the wife of a man with Parkinson's: "Doctor, my husband is a miracle—I have been praying his Parkinson's away and I think he will be the first person to be cured through prayer" (332). Dr. Jill does not directly confirm the cure: "I didn't really believe he would be cured. I couldn't dismiss the possibility either" (332). She then quotes with approval several more of her patients. Sam: "My belief in God and my associated faith in him have been and continue to be the most significant determining factor in the quality of my entire life" (333–34); Al: "Belief in God plays a big factor in just getting through the day and knowing he is always there for me" (340–41).

I have no problem with people crediting their religious faith or prayer with having a positive effect on their health, but I wonder if it is appropriate for a medical person, an expert in treating Parkinson's, to hint that a disease like Parkinson's can respond to deep faith and heartfelt prayers. People with Parkinson's have enough trouble answering the "Why me?" question. Can it help them to be told, even indirectly, that perhaps the reason for their diagnosis of Parkinson's and for their continuing decline as the disease progresses is that they do not pray often enough or believe deeply enough?

A6. *Parkinson's Disease and the Family*: *A New Guide*, by Nutan Sharma, MD, and Elaine Richman, PhD. Cambridge, Massachusetts: Harvard University Press, 2005. 222 pp.

> "It is far easier to think about and discuss assisted living and nursing home arrangements before they are needed."

The first sentence in the introduction to *Parkinson's Disease and the Family* explains the reference to family in the title: "Parkinson's disease is a chronic and progressive condition that affects not only the person with the disease but also his or her loved ones" (1). Much of the information about Parkinson's provided by the authors is pretty standard stuff. They present chapters on topics like diagnosing the disease, treatment options, finding help, intimacy, depression, dementia, clinical trials, and communicating with your treatment team. In this guide Drs. Sharma and Richman offer basic information about the disease, in admirably plain English, to both the frightened patients and their frightened family members.

The writing style is informal and chatty: "You may be wondering what put your relative or friend at risk for Parkinson's disease. Why Jack or Maria or Jennifer or Manuel? Why not Roberto or Dave or Cheryl?" (50) There is some use of numbers, but technical statistics are kept to a minimum: "More than 35 percent of people with advanced Parkinson's disease experience falls. Injuries tend to be minor cuts and bruises, but about 18 percent of falls result in the fracture of one or more bones" (64). That is good to know, but we search in vain for information about what percentage of those falls end in death.

The families of Parkinson's patients can't help but wonder how their relatives with the disease usually die, and when. I had hoped that the authors would say something about that sensitive subject. Like most writers of books about Parkinson's, they say almost nothing about dying. The closest they come is at the start of Chapter 13, "When Long-Term Arrangements Are Required": "Make it clear to all family members, preferably in writing as well as verbally, how you want to live and die" (170). Then, instead of saying any more about dying, and what the options are, the authors spin a story about Bill, a seventy-five-year-old man who has had Parkinson's disease for seventeen years. With the help of his seventy-two-year-old wife Sondra, he manages pretty well. But suddenly, one day, Sondra has a massive stroke and ends up in intensive care in a local hospital. She survives, but their three grown children are suddenly faced with decisions about what to do with Sondra and Bill. One of them wants their parents to move back to their home, where Bill can, with hired nurse-aide visits, look after Sondra. Others feel sure that Bill is not up to such responsibility and want to place them both in a nursing home. They talk with a social worker who helps them resolve the disagreement. What is the point of that little tale?

> The most important message is that it is far easier to think about and discuss assisted living and nursing home arrangements before they are needed. We recommend that the Parkinson's disease patient and all the members of the family who could be faced with decisions about a living situation address the issue early and as often as necessary. (173–74)

The last chapter, Chapter 14, "The Wedding," is an extended story about Jennifer, a young woman who is afraid to marry Rick, the man she loves, because her sixty-two-year-old father had been diagnosed with Parkinson's eight years earlier. She is worried that the disease is hereditary and that she is some sort of carrier who will bring into the world babies who will one day be diagnosed with Parkinson's. When she resolves that issue and plans the wedding, her father worries that he will stumble when he walks his daughter down the aisle and, after the wedding, when he dances with her. The story ends, of course, with everyone living happily ever after.

Would that all Parkinson's stories ended so happily!

A7. *Parkinson's Disease: 300 Tips for Making Life Easier* (second edition), by Shelley Peterman Schwartz. New York: Demos Medical Publishing, 2006. ix + 140 pp.

> "Exercise does not reverse or delay the symptoms of PD."

When one reads in the title of a 140-page book that it contains 300 tips for making life easier, it is easy to figure out that the book contains, on average, more than two tips per page. Actually, there are fewer than a

hundred pages of actual tips (the rest of the pages are taken up with lists
of resources, etc.). And there are actually 355 tips, not 300, so the actual
average number of tips per page is almost four. To put it another way, the
average length of each tip is about ten lines, or around three sentences.
To put it in still another way, readers of *Parkinson's Disease: 300 Tips for
Making Life Easier* should not expect great depth or complexity in the tips
being offered.

The tips are numbered from 1 to 355. By way of example, here are three
of them:

> **38. Keep a full set of duplicate keys in several places around the
> house**, in case you misplace a set. Always try to put the keys you
> regularly use in one designated place (say, in a dish or on a hook
> by the door most frequently used) to reduce the amount of time you
> spend hunting for them. (18)

> **49. If you plan to purchase new appliances**, consider buying a
> stove with a smooth top; it is much easier to clean. Select a side-
> by-side refrigerator/freezer, so that you can store both frozen and
> refrigerated items at eye level. (21)

> **85. Pour shampoo onto a sponge;** then rub the sponge on your
> hair. The shampoo is less likely to run into your eyes, and there's no
> chance of dropping a slippery bottle in the tub or shower. (36)

The first thing we might notice about these three tips is that none of
them is specific to people with Parkinson's disease. The advice may be
useful for anyone. That is all right, of course, but in a book with the title
Parkinson's Disease: 300 Tips for Making Life Easier one might have
assumed that the tips would be directed more specifically to people with
Parkinson's.

The second thing we might notice is that the advice may not be all
that wise. Is it really smart in these days of exploitation of the elderly and
infirm to encourage them to leave duplicate sets of keys lying around? We
have a smooth-top kitchen range, but I notice that Anne has to scrape the
brown crud off it with a razor blade several times a week. As for a side-by-
side refrigerator, why is it important to have our food at eye level? Is the
implication that the upper and lower shelves be kept empty? And is it really
good advice to squirt one's shampoo onto a sponge rather than onto one's
hair, or into one's hand? Will doing so really keep the shampoo out of our

eyes or keep us from dropping the bottle? Doesn't the sponge just give us something in addition to the bottle to hold, making it more likely that we will drop the bottle?

Shelley Schwartz does give some tips that are aimed specifically at people with Parkinson's. Here is what she says about the importance of exercise:

> **16. Make exercise part of your life.** Exercise does not reverse or delay the symptoms of PD, but it does help you make full use of your potential and improve your quality of life. (6)

I know of no one who would disagree with Shelley Schwartz that exercise needs to be part of the lives of people with Parkinson's, but I know many who would disagree that exercise does not delay the symptoms of the disease. People with Parkinson's have proved over and over that vigorous and repeated exercise does slow the disease down and does delay the symptoms.

There is lots of good general advice about "making life easier" for ourselves as we grow older, but we need keep in mind that Shelley Schwartz is not a doctor and does not have Parkinson's. She does have multiple sclerosis. While it is true that dealing with one progressive and incurable neurological disease gives her some authority to give tips to people with other progressive and incurable neurological diseases, you should be cautious. Take her advice if it makes sense to you and helps you, but trust your own instincts when you read a tip like this:

> **174. Keep an extra pair of pliers in the kitchen.** Use them to peel away the plastic seal from a jar of peanut butter, to pull the tab on a container of cream cheese, to grab the sealer strip from a can of frozen orange juice or a gallon of milk. (64)

It is good advice to have a pair of pliers close at hand in your kitchen, but peanuts and peanut butter, if taken with carbidopa/levidopa, keeps the medicine from reaching the brain in full strength. Parkinson's people are often warned against dairy products like milk and cream cheese. A writer more sensitive to the nutritional needs of people with Parkinson's would perhaps have picked different examples.

So here's my tip: if it is important to you to make your life "easier"— that is, to put the ease back into your *disease*—you will find some ideas worth testing in this book. If you want to make your life more meaningful, or more spiritual, or more helpful to others, you may perhaps want to look elsewhere.

A8. *Making the Connection between Brain and Behavior: Coping with Parkinson's Disease*, by Joseph H. Friedman, MD. New York: Demos Medical Publishing, 2007. xix + 193 pp.

> "While we use motor dysfunction to diagnose PD, it is actually the behavioral problems that cause the most devastating consequences of this illness."

The broad thesis of *Making the Connection between Brain and Behavior* is that while most neurologists, patients with Parkinson's, and their families have in the past thought of Parkinson's disease as a motor disease, it is more important to think of it as a behavioral disease. That is, we have tended to think of Parkinson's in terms of tremors, shuffling, stumbling, walking strangely, freezing, falling, balance, stiffness, lack of ability to swing the arms, slowness, stooping, walkers, and wheelchairs. Often far more troubling than those motor issues are the behavioral issues that can come with the disease: fatigue, nightmares, apathy, depression, anxiety, dementia, hallucinations, delusions, delirium, and various kinds of compulsive behavior such as buying, hoarding, hypersexuality, and pathological gambling.

In calling attention to these behavioral issues, Dr. Friedman draws on his two decades of caring for Parkinson's patients and talking with members of their families. Reading his book can be distressing. It is bad enough for people with Parkinson's to have to worry about the gradual physical deterioration that is our lot in life. Now we get to worry about the emotional and even psychotic changes that lurk around the bend. These can be worse—for ourselves and our families—than the motor issues:

> While we use motor dysfunction to diagnose PD, it is actually the behavioral problems that cause the most devastating consequences of this illness. It took me many years to recognize this, and when patients and families face these behavioral problems they feel

surprised and alone because they always thought that PD caused tremors, and not much else. Published studies have clearly shown that the most important problems causing nursing home placement of the PD patient is not slowness or the inability to walk. They are psychiatric. Similarly, the most stressful problem for caretakers are behavioral, not motor. (xv)

There is, of course, good news in the book. It is good news that none of us will demonstrate all of the behaviors that Dr. Friedman warns us of, that some of us will demonstrate none of the behaviors that he warns us of, and that some of the behaviors that he warns us of are readily treatable just by changing one or two of the medications we have been taking.

I found much to appreciate in Dr. Friedman's book. The short prologue entitled "No More Nagging," for example, helped me to understand that I am not alone in falling so often. I have always thought I was smart enough to learn from my mistakes. I have learned that I fall when I am going up an incline, or when I am walking on the grass, or when I am carrying something, or when I am talking to someone, or when I need to change direction, or when I approach a doorway or a gate, or when I am distracted by a cat or a flower. Why in the world do I not learn from my falls and not fall the next time? Dr. Friedman admits that he too is puzzled:

I don't know what to do when PD patients fall a lot. I have been impressed by how many PD patients fall in particular situations that they already know are problematic. Most patients fall when they try to turn and their feet stick to the ground. So, why don't they simply learn to cope with this by stopping, turning with a few small steps, or by leaning against a wall? I've asked some patients about this and I always get a shrug. I also hear from the caregiver that the patient is constantly being told, "Be careful. Turn slowly. Don't take your hands off the walker." Yet it happens daily or more. I used to say the same thing. "Stop and think before you turn."

One day I had a sudden insight. There are not many stronger stimuli for learning than a very bad experience. If you do something that results in a very bad outcome, you avoid doing that thing again. If you stick a fork in the socket you learn with a single experience never to do that again. Why is it that a PD patient who falls can do the same thing over and over again? I don't know, but I realized one day that if a fall won't teach a patient the danger, then my advice or a spouse's nagging isn't very likely to either.

What's the solution? I don't know. It's hard to keep from trying
to help. On the other hand, we must learn to avoid nagging. Nagging
is demoralizing for the nagger and the naggee. The nagger feels
ignored and the one being nagged feels misunderstood or weak, as if
not trying hard enough. (xviii–xix)

So I carry on, stupidly, falling when I go up an incline, when I walk on the
grass, when am distracted by a cat or a flower.

Dr. Friedman is to be commended for being sympathetic to the needs of
caregivers. In his Chapter 9, "Delusions," he talks about the most common
delusion of Parkinson's patients: accusing his or her spouse of infidelity:

While, of course, this may in fact be occurring, most of the time
these are groundless complaints that are frequently impossible
because the two are never out of sight of each other. […] Psychotic
symptoms are more stressful for caregivers than motor problems.
In fact, it has been recorded that caregiver stress is lower if the
patient is wheelchair bound and unable to provide much self-help
but is behaviorally intact, than if the patient is independent but has
behavior problems. I think there can be little so devastating to a
devoted spouse, having spent years in selfless effort to make life
better for their loved one, to then be accused of infidelity. That can
be the last straw. (97, 99)

Individual readers will find in Dr. Friedman's book answers to many
of their questions. Why are Parkinson's patients especially prone to
compulsive gambling (115–19)? Why do Parkinson's patients need to
urinate so often when they go to bed (128)? How do the families and
doctors of Parkinson's patients deal with the delicate issue of getting them
to give up driving (145–53)? Why should you hesitate before taking a
Parkinson's patient to the emergency ward (159–61)? And, of course, why,
despite the kind of evidence that Dr. Friedman presents here, do I continue
to think of Parkinson's disease as primarily a motor, not a behavioral,
disease? Is it because I stupidly keep falling down but have no delusions
about my wife's being unfaithful? I do *not* think she is having an affair with
the neighbor.

"Anne, where are you?" I do not *think* she is having an affair with the
neighbor.

"Hey, Anne? What are you doing?" *Could* she be having an affair with
the neighbor?

"Anne?"

Unfaithful bitch!

A9. *Parkinson's Disease: A Complete Guide for Patients and Families* (second edition), by William J. Weiner, MD, Lisa M. Shulman, MD, and Anthony E. Lang, MD. Baltimore: Johns Hopkins University Press, 2007. x + 278 pp.

> "[W]e understand that there are times when [patients] and their families feel hopeless, times when they feel desperate about their medical situation."

To live with Parkinson's disease is to live in a world of changes—changes in our symptoms, changes in our ability to cope, changes in our medication. The announced goal of the authors of *Parkinson's Disease* is to "contribute to a foundation of knowledge for persons who are living with Parkinson's disease in order to help them make healthy adjustments to these changes, to develop competency in self-monitoring and self-management, and to become effective partners in shared decision making with their physician" (xi). Those are noble goals, but this book does not fully achieve them.

The book is divided into five parts: I, "Introduction"; II, "Signs and Symptoms of Parkinson's Disease"; III, "Diagnosing Parkinson's Disease"; IV, "Treatment of Parkinson's Disease"; and V, "Other Issues." Of particular use are parts III and V.

Part III explains clearly the difficulty that physicians have in arriving at an accurate diagnosis. With few clinical, chemical, or electronic tools to help them, doctors must rely on their observation of the patient. They look for tremors, stiffness, slowness, gait, and balance problems. These symptoms are often not readily apparent early in the disease, and even when they are, can often indicate other diseases than Parkinson's.

Of particular interest in part V is the list of questions and answers in Chapter 18, the closing chapter. Among the questions are ones we have all wondered about but were reluctant to ask directly: What is the prognosis for someone with Parkinson's disease? Will I be an invalid? Will I still be able to drive my car? Will I be able to travel? Is it true that levodopa preparations work for only a limited period of time? As my disease progresses, will I be able to control my bladder and bowels? Is there sex after Parkinson's disease? Will I eventually require live-in help? Nursing home care? Will Parkinson's disease shorten my life?

Those seeking definite or encouraging answers in this book to such questions about the future will probably be disappointed. The three doctors who wrote this book generally give uncertain answers to most questions about what lies ahead or around the next corner: "The prognosis varies." "Parkinson's may seriously compromise your ability to drive safely." "For some people, yes, but not all." "Probably, but not always." "The disease follows a unique course in every individual." "Some people with Parkinson's [...]. On the other hand, many people with Parkinson's [...]."

Readers who seek encouraging news about what lies ahead should probably not read this book. Although the authors have much to say about drugs that can help to alleviate some symptoms, such readers will find the tone of the book to be overwhelmingly negative: "Parkinson's has neither a cure nor any treatment to slow down its progression" (4). "The central mechanism that controls muscle tone does not function adequately for the delicate interplay of muscles required to help us stand, walk, and balance. In addition, because Parkinson's disease also affects the autonomic nervous system (the largely unconscious system that controls our body temperature, digestive system, sexual function, and bladder control, among other functions), these systems may also act oddly" (9). "Although medications for Parkinson's disease may improve posture somewhat, no measure has been successful in preventing the development of this problem" (51). "Parkinson's disease is a progressive disorder. It continues to get worse" (61). "Parkinson's can cause a wide range of cognitive, behavioral, and psychiatric symptoms, and so can the drugs used to treat it" (77). "Although creating a brain lesion may help alleviate the symptoms of Parkinson's, surgery does not cure or even slow the disease: Parkinson's remains a degenerative disease: it continues to get worse" (211). "People with Parkinson's must understand that this procedure [deep brain stimulation] is no cure" (218–19).

To be sure, such statements are probably accurate enough, but are they really consistent with the stated goals of helping people who are living with Parkinson's make healthy adjustments as the disease progresses and to develop competency in self-monitoring and self-management? With so little to look forward to but more disability and increasing dependence, with so little encouragement to hope for a better future, what healthy adjustments are we to make?

If Parkinson's is bad as these three clinicians say it is, and if the future for people with Parkinson's is so dim, we might hope for at least a glimmer of human sympathy. We get a hint of it now and then in these pages, but often only to have it undermined, as in this section on alternative therapies for Parkinson's: "As physicians who see many patients with Parkinson's disease, we understand that there are times when they and their families feel hopeless, times with they feel desperate about their medical situation. In those moments, they may turn to alternative therapies, no matter how unrealistic or far-fetched they appear or how much they cost" (209). It is almost as if these three physicians want us to feel hopeless and desperate.

No, surely not.

A10. *Parkinson's Disease for Dummies*, by Michele Tagliati, MD, Gary N. Guten, MD, and Jo Horne. Hoboken, New Jersey: John Wiley and Sons, 2007. xvii + 363 pp.

> "Take charge of this thing—the same way you'd attack any other unlikely event (like losing your job or your home being damaged by fire). Life can hand you bigger problems than PD—really!"

Don't be put off by the title of this book, *Parkinson's Disease for Dummies*. It does not mean that only dummies get Parkinson's, or that only dummies should read this book about Parkinson's. It just means that the authors assume no special knowledge in their readers and so explain just about everything in simple and direct language. *Parkinson's Disease for Dummies* offers sensible, realistic, readable, and practical information about Parkinson's.

The three co-authors know and care a lot about this disease. Dr. Michele Tagliati teaches neurology at Mount Sinai School of Medicine and directs the Parkinson's Disease Center there. Dr. Gary Guten, an orthopedic surgeon with a specialty in sports medicine, was diagnosed with Parkinson's in 1995. Jo Horne is a writer whose sister has Parkinson's. Their collaboration brings together a wealth of knowledge, personal experience, and communication skills that provide an unusually useful resource for people who want—or suddenly need—to learn a lot about Parkinson's disease.

I cannot in a few pages do more than hint at the range of material covered in the twenty-four chapters, but I do want to give some sense of that range: recognizing early symptoms and later stages; reflecting on the possible causes of Parkinson's; locating a neurologist; coping with the diagnosis; denying your denial; channeling your anger, frustration, jealousies, sense of unfairness; telling (or not) your boss and your co-workers; protecting your income streams; purchasing (or not) long-term health insurance; understanding the Americans with Disabilities Act; understanding the role of complementary and alternative medicines, nutrition, acupuncture, and massage; making the most of the good years; confronting bravely the not-so-good years; managing family frictions; being sensitive to the needs and capabilities of your adult children; dealing with embarrassing things like intimacy, sexual dysfunction, urinary incontinence, and constipation; getting around voice and communication difficulties; deciding about traveling; volunteering for clinical trials; finding or creating a Parkinson's support group; coping with advanced Parkinson's; making your house safer; deciding whether, when, and where to move; getting your affairs and advanced directives in order; and so on.

I give here a sampling of the practical information and advice to be found in *Parkinson's Disease for Dummies*.

> **Acceptance.** "If you refuse to accept that PD is a fact of life for you, then you're wasting precious time and energy in denial. But, if you accept that most people get challenges in life and PD is yours, then you're ahead of the game" (11).

> **Causes.** "For the overwhelming number of patients who get Parkinson's, certain environmental factors seem to put the person at higher risk for getting the disease. [...] These factors include living in a rural area and using well water for drinking, cooking, and such" (21).

> **Choices.** "Understand that a PD diagnosis is not a death sentence. You have a life to live and choices to make about how you'll face each day, probably for years and even decades to come" (64).

> **Football.** "Think of PD as a 400-pound lineman constantly in

your face. He's there when you wake up and when you go to sleep. He gets in your way, blocking you when you try to work or play and when your friends come around. Sometimes he's well-behaved, maybe even sitting on the sidelines for awhile. But mostly he's charging, blocking, and even tackling to keep you from doing what you want" (69).

Fighting. "Thousands of PWP [People with Parkinson's] believe that a huge part of fighting PD is to approach it as only a piece of their lives. The point is this: Those facets of your life that defined you before you were diagnosed are still here—at least for the most part" (74–75).

Emergencies. "Stuff happens, and worst-case scenarios happen unexpectedly. Maybe you fall or burn yourself while preparing dinner and end up in the emergency room. Or, despite all precautions, you experience an adverse drug interaction that requires a stay in the hospital. Nonmedical emergencies—a fire, a weather event (such as a severe storm or tornado)—can also crop up. Our advice throughout this book is this: Have a plan in the event something unexpected happens. This doesn't mean you're assuming the worst. You just want to be ready—or as ready as possible" (82).

Hospital. "If you need to be admitted to the hospital, the cause isn't likely to be your PD. The more likely reason will be a serious injury (such as a hip fracture or head trauma from a fall) or another health condition (such as heart problems or diabetes). Regardless, be prepared with the necessary information" (85).

Humor. "We can't say this too often: An upbeat, optimistic attitude is one of your most effective weapons against PD. And right next to it the ability to laugh—with others, at yourself, and especially at your PD. We're talking black humor here, folks" (91).

Proactivity. "Take charge of this thing—the same way you'd attack any other unlikely event (like losing your job or your home being damaged by fire). Life can hand you bigger problems than PD—really! Unlike people facing a terminal illness, you have time and a reminder to be proactive and do what matters now, not someday. [...] There's nothing like a progressive illness to make you get off your butt, take that trip, write that novel, or go back to school" (104–05).

Water. "Flavor it with a slice of lemon or a little fruit juice if you can't take it straight, but six to eight big glasses every day. (And, no, soda, coffee, and tea don't count)" (153).

Exercise. "Exercising regularly boosts the power of neurotransmitters in your brain to enhance your mood and your ability to see life in a more positive light" (154).

Apathy. "The PWP's apathy can trigger frustration in family, friends, and the care partner. When those around an apathetic person begin to realize that they're working harder at fighting your PD than you are, the tendency is to think that the person suffering from apathy doesn't appreciate their efforts or help. The end result can be that family and friends gradually go back to their own lives, leaving the person with apathy (and the care partner) more isolated and in need of help than before" (187).

Adaptation. "Having Parkinson's is a life-changing situation— one that will continue to affect you for the rest of your days. But are you a PD patient, or are you still the same active, involved, in-charge person you were before you had PD? You can choose to allow a diagnosis of PD to dominate your daily routine even in the early stages or you can take the proactive approach—doing what it takes to adapt PD to your lifestyle" (224).

Most of the book is directed to the men and women who have Parkinson's. But I am happy to report that the authors are deeply sensitive to the special difficulties facing the families of these men and women, and particularly to the individuals—usually the spouses or adult children—who become care partners and, then, as the disease progresses, caregivers. Many of the chapters end with a word of advice to those who care for the people with Parkinson's. The authors provide a useful "Bill of Rights for the PD care partner" (288) and devote a whole chapter to "Ten Ways to Care for Your Care Partner" (329–32).

I quite like this book: it is well-written, practical, tough, respectful, funny, and affirming. It presents a consistent message: think positively, be upbeat, laugh, live for the present, and be kind to those around you. I am less of a dummy about Parkinson's disease than I was a week ago. You'd be a dummy not to give *Parkinson's Disease for Dummies* a read.

A11. *Parkinson's Disease: Reducing Symptoms with Nutrition and Drugs* (revised edition), by Geoffrey Leader, MD, and Lucille Leader. London: Denor Press, 2009. xiv + 165 pp.

> "Medical knowledge is constantly expanding. [...] Patient individuality makes it imperative for supervision by healthcare professionals at all times."

After reading a book like this, we cannot help but be impressed—no, distressed—with just how complex Parkinson's disease is. It takes thirty-four chapters to explain the many and varied bits of nutritional information we need to have at our fingertips if we want to stay healthy, more or less. Here are just ten of the chapter titles, selected because they are short (only one or two words long): 3, "Body Composition"; 12, "Compromised Liver"; 13, "Food Intolerance"; 14, "Food Additives"; 15, "Free Radicals"; 16, "Environmental Hazards"; 20, "Weight Control"; 21, "Parasites"; 30, "Dental Health"; 32, "Improving Sleep." The other chapter titles are longer, such as 22, "Improving Bowel Environment after Antibiotics."

In a short review I cannot mention more than a few of the bits of information and advice the authors give. I select below some topics and statements that I found interesting.

> **Recommended snacks**: "Almonds and other nuts (not peanuts or cashews which may contain mycotoxins), together with fruit, are a good combination" (14).

> **Constipation**: "The most effective [high fiber foods] for people with Parkinson's disease seem to be prunes (which have been soaked overnight) and thereafter figs. It is not sufficient to take one serving only per day. Prunes and figs should be taken in small quantities spread over the whole day" (28).

Mercury: "It is not recommended for all Parkinson's disease patients to automatically have their mercury fillings removed. This process in itself can be detrimental to that detoxification" (63).

Water: "It is vital to drink eight-to-ten glasses of fluid daily to facilitate bowel movement" (77, see also 79 and 85, where the advice is repeated).

Raw meats: "It may be prudent to choose only cooked foods in restaurants. Parasites can be found in inadequately washed salads, raw meat, fish" (90).

Depression: "Depression and stress often affect people with Parkinson's disease. This can be due to the illness itself as dopamine metabolizes (is converted) to noradrenaline and adrenaline. However, it would be unnatural if people were not feeling depressed at having developed this disease" (131).

Humor: "Laughter therapy (comedy videos, joke books), avoiding depressing subjects" (134).

Sexuality: "In some cases, people who develop a movement disorder, such as Parkinson's disease, are embarrassed by their movement disturbance—and so they withdraw! This is not because their feelings for their partners have waned. Sometimes, it is because they doubt their partners' continued feelings for them, in view of new mental, physical, practical, and emotional adjustments that may be necessary. [...] Apart from sexual intercourse and outercourse (intimacy without penetration), there are other successful ways to give personal assurances of one's continued recognition and affection—regular hugs and words of love work wonders" (139).

The authors do not, of course, promise that following their multifaceted advice will make people with Parkinson's well. They are careful to suggest only that following their advice may reduce some of our symptoms. They are careful to insist that people with Parkinson's act only on the advice of someone on their own healthcare team:

The recommendations in this book are not intended to replace general medical advice or the advice of a neurologist, nutritionist, dietician, clinical biochemist, pathologist, pharmacist, psychologist, surgeon, anesthetist, dentist, occupational therapist, nurse, physiotherapist, exercise therapist or any other healthcare professional. (iv)

That is an appalling list of the health-care professionals we are supposed to consult (and pay for!) before we take any action. And if that is not daunting enough, the disclaimer goes on to tell us that the information in the book may well be out of date anyhow, and besides, it may not apply to individual readers because all individuals are, well, individual:

> Medical knowledge is constantly expanding. As new clinical experience and experimental knowledge is gained, management needs to be constantly re-evaluated and updated. Patient individuality makes it imperative for supervision by healthcare professionals at all times. (iv)

The obvious question is this: Why should we read this book at all if we are to be sent back to individual consultations with expensive medical professionals anyhow? There are different ways to answer that question. One is that the authors and the publisher want to avoid legal liability if someone sues them for giving advice that turns out to be misleading, outdated, ineffective, or harmful. Another answer is that people with Parkinson's need to be aware that what they eat, drink, and do *can* make a difference in how they feel, how they manage their disease, how their caregivers get along, and how long they live. Still another is that a book like this can give readers the basic information and vocabulary so that they are in a position to ask intelligent questions the next time they see their neurologists (primary care physicians, physical therapists, dentists, psychiatrists, or whoever).

My own favorite chapter is Chapter 34, "The Carer's Guide," which gives full recognition to the importance of the caregiver, as we usually call them in the USA, or care partners. I like the British term better, if only because the people we are speaking of are important less because they give care than because they simply *care*. The authors of *Parkinson's Disease: Reducing Symptoms with Nutrition and Drugs* are fully aware of the vital role the carers play in ensuring that the many and confusing suggestions in their book are implemented. These include knowing which foods will least interfere with the optimal efficacy of pharmaceutical medications, when to eat so as to reduce dyskinesia, which foods and fluids can promote intestinal regularity, and so on. This chapter makes wise suggestions about the personal rights of the carers, the need to care for themselves as well as for their charges, the necessity for frequent respite, how to deal with their own anger and grief at the hand that fate has dealt them, how to handle the unremitting stress and frustration of long-term caring. Chapter 34 has important advice, such as: "Count the blessings that you still have and appreciate yourself as a worthy and loving human being who is capable of a very special job," "Do something loving towards yourself each day," and "Attend activities at caregivers' support groups" (147). To those I would add, "Try to remember that the person you care for cares for you, appreciates all that you do, and would eagerly do anything to make your life more pleasant."

A12. *Natural Therapies for Parkinson's Disease,* by Dr. Laurie K. Mischley. Seattle: Coffeetown Press, 2010. 163 pp.

> "It doesn't taste nearly as bad as many people think it might!"

Laurie K. Mischley, ND, PhD, is a Seattle-based naturopathic doctor, one of several professionals who make up Seattle Integrative Medicine on Roosevelt Avenue in the University District. She also has had faculty appointments at Bastyr University and at the University of Washington, where she recently earned her PhD. For fifteen years she has been treating patients with Parkinson's disease. Because of her experience with patients and her increasing involvement in research, she is convinced that people with Parkinson's can be helped by both traditional and nontraditional therapies.

In *Natural Therapies for Parkinson's Disease*, Dr. Mischley calls for the integration of the conventional approach to Parkinson's—involving carbidopa-levodopa, agonists, and other pharmaceuticals—with the naturopathic approach—involving nutrition and vitamin supplements. She is convinced that if neurologists and naturopaths work together, then patients need not assume that Parkinson's is always progressive or that it can never be slowed, halted, or even reversed.

Conventional therapies, she says, are good at "defense." They treat the disease once it manifests itself through its most common symptoms: tremor, slowness, gait, and balance. Conventional therapies ease the symptoms by using pharmaceuticals to reduce the symptoms once they show up—which is typically a decade after the brain begins to lose the ability to create dopamine.

Naturopathic therapies, on the other hand, she says, are good at "offense." Their role is preventing the symptoms from showing up in the first place and then, if they do appear, working to stop, slow, or reverse the progression of the disease. Dr. Mischley insists that to succeed, a patient needs to have both an aggressive offense and a strong defense.

How, in practical terms, can the offense go into action to head off the arrival of the symptoms? Her answer is that there are some early warning signals. For example, if you have a close relative who had Parkinson's, your chances of getting the disease are much higher. If you were in Vietnam when we were using Agent Orange as a defoliant, or if you grew up drinking well water or spring water in a rural community where farmers used pesticides and herbicides, then you might want to heed the advice that Dr. Mischley gives in her book.

What is that advice? Well, some of it is pretty technical. Dr. Mischley says in her introduction that her book can be used by "patients, physicians, caregivers, and relatives of those with Parkinson's." (1). When she talks about Lewy bodies she apparently has in mind an audience of physicians: "Lewy bodies are composed of alpha-synuclein and ubiquitin, two proteins associated with disease progression in PD. [...] They are found floating in the cytoplasm of neurons" (11). Yeah, right. Few patients will know what in the world she is saying. In a sense, however, it does not matter whether lay people can understand technical sentences like that, but it is comforting to us to know that she does. She needs to understand why she gives the advice she gives; we need to understand only what the advice is.

What are free radicals? I don't know. I gather from reading her book that all human brains produce bad guys called free radicals, which tend to destroy brain tissue. In healthy brains these free radicals are offset by good guys called antioxidants. In the brains of people with Parkinson's, however, the antioxidants are not strong enough or numerous enough to kill off the bad guys. All we really need to know about free radicals is that by eating beans and blueberries we can improve our chances of successfully doing battle with them.

In the rest of this short review I list some of the advice that Dr. Mischley gives to people with Parkinson's and people with a family history of Parkinson's who want to give themselves the best chance of avoiding it:

What to drink

—Tea or coffee.
—Wine or beer in moderation.
—Filtered water, and plenty of it.

What not to drink

—Milk.
—Well water in agricultural areas where farmers use pesticides.

What to eat

—Vegetables, fruits, and nuts.
—Orange and red vegetables like carrots, bell peppers, and apricots.
—Poultry.
—Fish.
—Organically-grown foods.
—Nutrient-rich foods (see pp. 60–61 for an alphabetical list, from Artichokes to Zucchini, of nearly a hundred of these).

What not to eat

—Dairy products (butter, cheese, ice cream, yogurt).
—Pork.
—Beef.

What else to avoid

—Exposure to aluminum, which is used as an additive in some processed cheeses, baked goods, and grain products. Do not drink liquids packaged in aluminum cans.
—Overeating: "If your belly is bigger than your hips, you're probably eating too much, and the wrong things, too" (57).
—Shade: Direct sunshine on your skin is a good source of vitamin B12.

Dr. Mischley has things to say also about the following:

—**Carnitine**—"If you don't eat meat, you should take a carnitine supplement" (63).

—**Chelation**—"The act of removing metals from the body" (65).

—**Cholesterol**—"If possible, avoid the use of statins as cholesterol lowering agents" (69).

—**Choline**—"Indicated for individuals looking to reduce their dose of levodopa" (75).

—**Constipation**—If you don't have at least one bowel movement a day, you are dangerously constipated: "The bowels are one of the primary routes of eliminating unwanted waste and dangerous byproducts. When stool sits in the colon, the toxicants are reabsorbed into the bloodstream and recirculated throughout the body" (80). Take in enough liquid and fiber to achieve two bowel movements a day.

—**Curcumin**—"Use turmeric liberally! Add it to scrambled eggs, chicken, and vegetables" (87).

—**Fish oil**—Take it in liquid rather than in capsule form: "It doesn't taste nearly as bad as many people think it might!" (94).

Dr. Mischley devotes a chapter to recommendations for the children of people with Parkinson's: "A family history of PD is the single strongest predictor of developing this disease. [...] The cure for Parkinson's is prevention. Loss of smell and constipation may be early symptoms. [...] The earlier one gets started on the task of preventing and slowing the disease, the better. [...] I recommend that all children of PD parents avoid dairy. [...] I recommend that all children of PD parents drink more green tea" (137–38).

Excuse me. I need to run out and ask my four adult children about how often they poop and whether they can still smell it. No, not really, but I will buy them each a box of green tea and a copy of *Natural Therapies for Parkinson's Disease*.

A13. *100 Questions and Answers about Parkinson Disease* (second edition), by Abraham N. Lieberman, MD. Sudbury, Massachusetts: Jones and Bartlett Publishers, 2011. xi + 262 pp.

> "Parkinson seems more difficult to conquer because, unlike the other diseases, we don't know the cause, but our technology is more advanced than in 1900, our doctors better trained, and our resources greater: I believe a cure will come—and in our lifetime."

Dr. Abraham Lieberman, director of the Muhammad Ali Parkinson Center in Phoenix, has studied, taught, researched, and written about Parkinson's disease for more than four decades. When I saw the title of this book, I was curious to know how many of the questions that I personally wanted answers to would actually be answered in a book called *100 Questions and Answers about Parkinson Disease*. Before I read the book I jotted down five questions I had about Parkinson's disease: a) What causes Parkinson's? b) Why has my voice grown weaker and my stutter gotten worse since I was diagnosed with Parkinson's? c) When my feet "freeze," what can I do to keep from falling? d) Is it true what I've been told over and over, that you don't die *of* Parkinson's, but you die *with* it? e) Are we any closer to a cure for Parkinson's than we were a decade ago?

a) What causes Parkinson's? Dr. Lieberman asks and answers seven related questions: 4) What causes Parkinson Disease? 5) What puts me at risk for developing Parkinson disease? 6) Is Parkinson disease inherited? 7) Do toxins in the environment cause Parkinson disease? 8) Can a head injury or boxing cause Parkinson disease? 9) Do strokes cause Parkinson disease? 10) Do viruses cause Parkinson disease? I grew up and spent most of my life in rural Pennsylvania, where I drank well water, so I was especially interested in his answer to his question 7) Do toxins in the environment cause Parkinson disease?: "There are, literally, hundreds of thousands of potential toxins in the air, the soil, in your home, at your work, and in your food and water. Whether any given toxin causes PD has not yet been clinically proven" (15).

b) Why has my voice grown weaker and my stutter gotten worse since I was diagnosed with Parkinson's? I checked the index under "voice," "speaking," and "stuttering" but found no entries for any of them. Later, as I read the book, I found a question that had apparently escaped the indexer: 19) Is difficulty speaking part of Parkinson disease? Dr. Lieberman's answer is yes:

> About half of all PD patients have difficulty speaking. […] For most PD patients, voice difficulty manifests as a decrease in loudness, tone, and pitch. Your voice may be described as low, monotonous, and unvarying. Voice difficulty in PD, like difficulty moving, arises because the muscles involved in speaking are affected: they become rigid, they move slowly and incompletely. (59–60)

Dr. Lieberman says nothing about stuttering.

    c) When my feet "freeze," what can I do to keep from falling? Dr. Lieberman asks this question: *33) What is freezing of gait (FOG)?* Dr. Lieberman reports that FOG occurs "in 30% of PD patients with advanced PD," but he does not mention falling as a danger associated with FOG. He gives some "tricks" that have helped some people dealing with FOG: pretend you are stepping over an imaginary line; use a cane outfitted with laser light; hum a tune or chant a phrase like "Go, Go, Go." He mentions these as a way to start walking if you are frozen, not as a way to prevent falling. In his answer to the next question, *34) Why do I fall?* Dr. Lieberman talks about falling as a balance problem, not a freezing problem. He gives advice about avoiding wet, icy, and uneven surfaces and walking in dark places. That is good advice, of course, but it does not precisely answer my question. For me, falling results when my body leans forward a bit as if I were about to take a step, but my feet say, "not this time, pal," and down I go. Avoiding slippery and poorly lit places will not help me because I mostly freeze and fall in dry, well-lighted places.

    d) Is it true what I've been told over and over, that you don't die *of* Parkinson's, but you die *with* it? It has always struck me as at best evasive, at worst false, to say that Parkinson's won't kill you. If a man with Parkinson's stumbles while crossing a street and is run down by a truck, is it really accurate to say he was killed by a truck, not by the Parkinsonian freezing that caused his stumble? If a bedridden woman gets bed sores that become infected, is it really fair to say she died of infected bed sores rather than of the Parkinson's that put her in bed? If a man with Parkinson's has trouble swallowing, gets water in his lungs, and winds up with pneumonia, is it fair to say that he died of pneumonia, not Parkinson's? My question coincides nicely with Dr. Lieberman's question *12) Can I die from*

Parkinson disease? Here is his answer: "Do people die of PD? Technically not. But PD sets the body up for death. Whether patients die of PD, or from PD complications, they die. The remedy is research to find the cause of PD or slow its progression so patients can outlive its consequences" (35). That answer leads directly to my fifth question.

    e) Are we any closer to a cure for Parkinson's than we were a decade or two ago? That is similar to Dr. Lieberman's last question: *100) When will there be a cure?* His answer bears quoting:

> Although the cause or causes of PD are unknown, much is known about how specific substances injure cells in the brain including the dopamine cells. And, since the introduction of levodopa and the dopamine agonists, much has been learned about how the brain works. [...] PD cannot yet be cured, but its rate of progression may be slowed. [...] In 1900, people with tuberculosis, syphilis, or polio asked the same questions as people with PD today ask: When will there be a cure? The answer was then as now—I don't know, but I'm confident it'll come. As surely as we conquered tuberculosis, syphilis, and polio, we'll conquer PD. Parkinson seems more difficult to conquer because, unlike the other diseases, we don't know the cause, but our technology is more advanced than in 1900, our doctors better trained, and our resources greater: I believe a cure will come—and in our lifetime. (235–36)

That seems a very vague answer. What does Dr. Lieberman mean by "in our lifetime"? Whose lifetime?

    Are Dr. Lieberman's hundred questions ones you care about, ones you want to know his answers to? Probably, yes, most of them. Is his book the kind of book in which you can expect to find answers to the questions you want to ask? Perhaps, but you will find both his questions and his answers to be generic. If you want to know in general about Parkinson's, you will learn a lot from Dr. Lieberman. If you want to know in particular about your own health and your own best options, you will be better off asking your own neurologist.

A14. *Pioneers of Recovery: Stories of Nine Pioneers Who Reversed the Symptoms of Parkinson's Disease* (second edition), by **Robert Rodgers, PhD. Parkinson's Recovery, 2012. 245 pp.**

> "Listen to your body as you read each chapter. Use your own intuition and judgment to decide whether the therapy or approach being discussed is something you might want to investigate further."

Cheryl had a dentist insert an implant in her mouth to alleviate her Parkinson's symptoms. Lidia Epp found a connection between her ex-husband's Parkinson's disease and her own skin condition called Candida. Lexie found that taking low doses of Naltrexone improved her symptoms substantially. Sharry Edwards used acoustics and bio-frequencies in a tone-box to reduce the symptoms of Parkinson's. Howard Shifke treated his Parkinson's by using traditional Chinese chants and exercises to cleanse his liver, and used various holistic medical practices to pave the way for his body to cure itself of the disease. Nan Little found that strenuous physical activity, especially biking and mountaineering, helped to alleviate her Parkinson's symptoms. Gord Summer used massage and what he called the "Power of the Mind" to keep himself calm enough to stay engaged and optimistic. Bianca found that the practice of the Chinese art of Qigong helped energy flow through her body and permitted her to reduce or eliminate her Parkinson's symptoms. Daniel Loney discovered that the regular practice of Tai Chi eliminated some of his Parkinson's symptoms altogether and greatly reduced others.

What do these nine brave men and women have in common? According to Robert Rodgers, who is quick to point out that he is not a medical doctor but an ex-college professor, "the nine pioneers confronted debilitating symptoms of Parkinson's disease and each recovered using an approach that was uniquely suited to their situation" (16).

Rodgers does not single out any of the nine approaches as being especially worthy of imitation or emulation: "If you decide to pursue any one of the therapies presented here, you may be either shocked to discover your symptoms vanish so quickly or frustrated to discover that the therapy is a waste and offers no relief whatsoever" (17). He does not claim to have researched any of the nine approaches. Indeed, he says, if you want to wait for them to be evaluated scientifically before you try them, "please plan on living 200 more years. You may need to extend your time on earth to 300 years" (19). Why can we expect no corroborating research? Because medical research is paid for by pharmaceutical companies seeking not to find a cure but to increase their own profits by finding expensive ways to treat the symptoms of Parkinson's: "Who is going to fund research to evaluate a therapy that is natural, safe, and has no side effects? Such is the case with most of the therapies presented in this book. Such therapies do not offer profit potential for any company" (20).

How, then, are you to know which, if any of these therapies may be the right one for you? "I do not have a clue," Rodgers says, "what therapy would be best for you to pursue" (21). It is up to you to do your own research:

> Who has the "right" answer for you? Whose advice can you trust? There is only one source of reliable information. The one and only person who can figure out what you need to do to recover is—you. Your body knows the answer—just ask. [...] Only certain therapies and modalities will be right for you. Which therapy or approach covered here appeals to you? Which chapter do you feel a surge of energy when you read it? Listen to your body as you read each chapter. Use your own intuition and judgment to decide whether the therapy or approach being discussed is something you might want to investigate further. Trust your own intuition and you will always make good decisions. (18–19)

Statements like that will sound to some readers like an abdication of authorial responsibility. If readers are to be thrown back on their own individual intuition and get no help from the man who selected these nine pioneers for attention, why buy the book in the first place? Indeed, why read any of the chapters if the man who presents them does not himself believe that a cure for Parkinson's is possible for anyone who now has the disease:

> There will never be a single cure for persons who currently experience the symptoms for Parkinson's. You may be thinking at this point—shucks! That is why I bought this book. The causes are complex and multifaceted. You will be profoundly disappointed if you are hoping that a single, simple "cure" of any form—including

pills or surgeries —will soon be discovered. Pills and surgeries mask symptoms. They do not address the underlying cause of the symptoms. (17)

Rodgers does not address the underlying cause of the symptoms, either.

I put down *Pioneers of Recovery: Stories of Nine Pioneers Who Reversed the Symptoms of Parkinson's Disease* with a sense that too many questions remained unanswered. How can we be sure, for example, that all nine of these "pioneers" really had Parkinson's disease and not some other condition that looked like Parkinson's disease? Rodgers admits, after all, that he is "not qualified to diagnose or treat Parkinson's disease" (21). How valid is the undigested and unverified radio-talk-show testimony of individuals who believed that they had found an approach that relieved some of their symptoms? What are the implications of Rodgers's statement that the radio interviews were "heavily edited" (16) for the book? What was left out or put in?

How much can we learn from a researcher who shies away from research: "my job as a researcher is to identify the many wonderful options that are available and to alert everyone with Parkinson's disease that recovery is possible" (21). What does Dr. Rodgers mean in the subtitle to his book that these nine "reversed" the symptoms of the disease? What does he mean by "recovery"? When he says that the nine pioneers "recovered" from "the debilitating symptoms of Parkinson's disease" (16), that sounds like they found a permanent cure. But the stories themselves do not always bear that out, and Rodgers himself qualifies that assertion by stating that "some pioneers are symptom free today. Others have a few symptoms that flare up from time to time. But, they too have recovered significantly" (16). When he tells his readers, "If you want to recover you can" (21), what precisely does Rodgers mean by "recover" in that statement? Does he mean "recover" or "recover significantly"? And, whatever he means, is it really fair for him to imply that people who do not recover fail only because they do not "want to"? Don't we have enough burdens to bear without being invited to believe that our failure to recover from Parkinson's is our own fault?

A15. *Navigating Life with Parkinson Disease,* by Sotirios A. Parashos, MD, PhD, Rose Wichmann, PT, and Todd Melby. New York: Oxford University Press, 2013. xx + 293 pp.

> "There is general optimism among Parkinson disease specialists that drugs that treat the disease itself, not just its symptoms, and even a cure may not be that far off."

The nautical title of *Navigating Life with Parkinson Disease* is fitting. To be told that we have Parkinson's or to find ourselves caring for or about someone who has Parkinson's is to embark on a journey into strange seas. This book is designed to help us find our way in what are for most of us uncharted waters. The preface claims that the book aims to be "a good compass" to "the basics of Parkinson's, the theories about its causes, the symptoms of is various stages, and the available treatments, including medications, therapies, and brain surgery" (xix-xx). The book, endorsed by the American Academy of Neurology, accomplishes those aims. It will be especially helpful to the newly diagnosed and to their partners, family members, friends, and colleagues.

In fourteen chapters, the authors of *Navigating Life with Parkinson Disease* answer such questions as: What is Parkinson's disease? What causes it? What are the four major symptoms that neurologists look for in diagnosing the disease? How will the disease change our lives? What "weapons" will help us fight back? When should we start taking levodopa? How can we manage specific symptoms like tremor, slowness, rigidity, balance, freezing, fatigue, dyskinesia, drooling? What are some of the problems that may lie ahead for us, problems with speech, vision, bladder control, constipation, cognition, loss of mobility, sleep, impulsive behavior, anxiety, sexuality, depression, and so on. What should we do about driving, traveling, involvement in research? Can exercise, music, dance, spirituality help us? How can we help our care partners stay healthy? What are some of the practical plans we should make for the future—things like "personal affairs," "arrangements," "powers of attorney," "trusts," and "directives"?

To raise such questions, of course, is to risk alienating us with page after page of reminders that we have a disease with no cure, a disease that gets only worse, a disease that makes steady inroads into our independence. We all know that growing old with Parkinson's is no bundle of joy. The authors of *Navigating Life with Parkinson Disease* are to be commended for not trying to shield us from the truth about what lies ahead: "Being diagnosed with a chronic illness is frightening. It's natural to focus on how Parkinson disease will make life worse. Undoubtedly life will present a person living with Parkinson's with many challenges every step of the way, and feelings of despair, disappointment, loss, and being overwhelmed may often darken one's perception of life" (85).

But this book is, finally, about pursuing a wise life with Parkinson's, not about preparing for an early end of life because of Parkinson's. The authors make every effort to persuade us not to be merely angry that we have a dreaded disease, but also to be grateful that we have it now, not a few decades ago before discoveries of levodopa and deep brain stimulation added bonus years to our functional lives as people with Parkinson's. They give us strategies that have helped others deal with the disease: humor, spirituality, joining support groups, getting exercise, joining a health club, taking up group singing or dancing. And they give us hope that things may get better: "There is general optimism among Parkinson disease specialists that drugs that treat the disease itself, not just its symptoms, and even a cure may not be that far off" (32).

The authors provide useful, honest, and clearly-stated advice. They use technical terms when they need to but are careful to give definitions that most of us will be able to comprehend. Some of these terms we need to understand to make sense of our disease, and some we will need to understand so that we can talk with and understand the various medical practitioners we will encounter on our voyage with Parkinson's: blood-brain barrier, COMT inhibitors, deep brain stimulation, diplopia, dopamine receptors, micrographia, neurodegenerative, neuroprotective, neurotransmitter, orthostatic hypotension, postural instability, substantia nigra. Such terms are defined not only along the way but also in a composite glossary at the end (see pages 261–71).

Particularly engaging are the little personal bits of advice in boxes called "Ask the Experts." For example, Susan Imke, GPN-D, gives a two-page answer (193–95) to the question, "What should I watch or change in my diet?" The last chapter, "Planning for Your Future: Managing Your Personal Affairs," written by two lawyers, Murray Sagsveen and Laurie Hanson, offers advice that will prove useful for anyone wanting to provide a smooth transition to the port that lies just over the western horizon.

Sure, there are some rough seas ahead, but *Navigating Life with*

Parkinson Disease will help us to sail them with skill, confidence, grace, and courage.

A16. *Parkinson's Treatment: Ten Secrets to a Happier Life,* by Michael S. Okun, MD. Copyright 2013 by Michael S. Okun. xi + 118 pp.

> "[T]he hidden path toward hope and happiness, [...] the 'secrets' that may lead to hope and a happier life, [...] the core values necessary to achieve happiness despite chronic disease."

Dr. Michael S. Okun has excellent credentials. He teaches, does research, and publishes articles about Parkinson's disease. He was one of the first research grant recipients at the Michael J. Fox Foundation. He co-directs the Center for Movement Disorders and Neurorestoration at the University of Florida. He is the National Medical Director of the National Parkinson's Foundation. He is in demand as a speaker at hospitals, universities, and conferences around the world. When such a man publishes a list of "ten secrets to a happier life" for people with Parkinson's we should all pay attention. Who among us would not want to know such secrets? Who among us would not want to get ourselves on track to a happier life?

The subtitle of *Parkinson's Treatment* claims that the ten secrets will lead to a happier life. That claim is repeated several times in the author's introduction: "helping map a road to a *happier* and more meaningful life, [...] the hidden path toward hope and *happiness*, [...] the spark to ignite the light of hope that will help to guide to a destination that includes a *happier* and more meaningful life, [...] the 'secrets' that may lead to hope and a *happier* life, [...] the core values necessary to achieve *happiness* despite chronic disease, [...] hope leads to *happiness* and happiness will lead to a meaningful life" (viii–x, italics added).

So, what are the ten secrets that will lead to happiness? Dr. Okun tells us that when we hear the four dreaded words, "You have Parkinson's disease," we should do these ten things: 1) make sure it really is Parkinson's disease and not Alzheimer's, or ALS (Lou Gehrig's disease), or a brain tumor, or a stroke; 2) take our medicines on time; 3) find out whether deep brain stimulation (DBS) is a good option for us; 4) seek treatment if we feel anxious or depressed; 5) get adequate sleep; 6) be aware that some

Parkinson's medicines can cause addiction-like compulsive behaviors such as gambling, hoarding, and watching pornography; 7) get regular exercise; 8) be prepared ahead of time for possible stays in a hospital; 9) keep informed about new medicines and treatments for Parkinson's; 10) stay optimistic so that we can have, despite our Parkinson's, a full, happy, and meaningful life.

Few of us will disagree with those ten pieces of advice. They reflect well enough our own experience with Parkinson's. But are these really "secrets"? A secret is something that is concealed from others, something that only a few privileged people know about. There is nothing really secret about that list. Many books about Parkinson's say the same things. If almost any movement disorder specialist, almost any Parkinson's patient with a year or two of experience, would know about most or all of those secrets, are they really secrets?

Once we get past the hype about the "secrets" and the "hidden path" to happiness, Dr. Okun's book has much to recommend it. The advice it gives about not confusing Parkinson's with other neurological conditions, about taking our meds at the right times, about the possibility of making our brain electric through DBS, about reporting depression to our doctors, about getting enough sleep—that advice is helpful and well-stated. Certainly it is wise for people with Parkinson's to know about the dangers of compulsive behavior that certain medicines can bring on, about the advantages of regular exercise, about what to expect (and not expect) when we are hospitalized.

Let's consider Chapter 8, "Be Prepared for Hospitalization." Dr. Okun tells us that few hospitals are really prepared to take care of Parkinson's patients. The staff often do not know how important it is to follow the patient's medication schedule, and do not know that certain drugs are particularly dangerous for patients with Parkinson's. Dr. Okun recommends that Parkinson's patients prepare in advance a hospital kit with such items as these: a bracelet identifying the wearer as having Parkinson's, a Parkinson's fact sheet, the neurologist's name and contact information, a current medications list with a detailed medication schedule, and a supply of medications. He recommends that a family member become an active advocate for the patient. That is all excellent advice, but is it really a "Parkinson's treatment" and is it really a "secret to a happier life"?

Dr. Okun is especially good at telling stories about what his patients have taught him, about the history of Parkinson's, and about what current medical researchers around the world are finding out. *Parkinson's Treatment: Ten Secrets to a Happier Life* will find its best audience among the newly diagnosed, the men and women—and their friends and families—who have just heard the four troubling words, "You have Parkinson's disease." Will the secrets that Dr. Okun reveals to these people, the hidden path he shows them, make them happy? Probably not. But happiness is perhaps not a realistic goal for readers of a book like this.

Parkinson's Treatments: Ten Secrets to a Happier Life, may do something more important than deliver happiness. For the newly diagnosed, it may begin the process of understanding what this disease is all about. It may give those who have Parkinson's the tools to help them face courageously, empathetically, and cheerfully the good years that lie ahead.

A17. *Understanding Parkinson's Disease: A Self-Help Guide* (second edition), by David L. Cram, MD, Steven H. Schechter, MD, and Xiao-Ke Gao, MD. Omaha, Nebraska: Addicus Books, 2013. viii + 148 pp.

> "Self-help is a positive approach to your condition that says. 'I have power. I have responsibility. I can make a difference in my disease'."

Two of the three doctors who collaborated on *Understanding Parkinson's Disease* had personal reasons for wanting to write a book like this. Dr. Cram, by training a dermatologist who specialized in psoriasis, was diagnosed with Parkinson's in 1991. He died in 2009. Dr. Gao, originally from Beijing, became interested in neurology in part because her mother had lived with the disease for some thirty years. Dr. Schechter is a neurologist in Michigan.

Their slender book was designed particularly for people newly diagnosed with Parkinson's, their families, and their friends, all of whom would naturally tend to focus on the negatives of the disease: it is chronic, it is progressive, it is debilitating, it is incurable. There are some medicines that can treat some of the symptoms for awhile, and there are some surgeries that can help some of the people with the disease. The medicines, however, can have unpleasant side effects and the surgeries are risky. Neither the medicines nor the surgeries can give more than temporary relief. The disease grinds on and on eating away at the brain. Given those well-known facts about the disease, it is easy to feel discouraged and helpless. The thesis of *Understanding Parkinson's Disease* is that while it is easy "to feel overwhelmed or believe there is nothing you can do, [...], there is plenty you can do to improve your life or that of someone you love" (1).

> **Chapter 1, A Self-Help Approach to Parkinson's Disease**, lays out the essential thesis of the book: "Self-help is a positive approach to your condition that says. 'I have power. I have responsibility. I can make a difference in my disease'." Successful self-help, they tell us, depends on four qualities: 1) **Attitude:** "We do know that a positive attitude can improve the quality of your life. It can make you feel better. It can also enable you to take the self-help steps you need to keep feeling as good as you can for as long as you can"; 2) **Knowledge:** "Equipping yourselves with knowledge will reduce your fears and enable you to make the best-informed medical choices"; 3) **Partnership with Your Doctors:** "Self-help does not mean doing everything by and for yourself. [...] Your doctors must select the right medicine in the correct dosage for your symptoms. Your job is to take the right amount of medication on time, keep track of your symptoms and side effects, let the doctors know how the medication is working, and report any problems you may be having with the treatment regimen"; 4) **Taking Action:** "Taking action means doing the things that make you feel better, slow the disability, and keep you independent for as long as possible" (1–3).

Like much of the rest of the book, these four qualities seem simple and obvious. Do we really think, even shortly after diagnosis, that a negative attitude is good for us, that knowledge is bad for us, that we don't need to listen to or communicate with our doctors, or that we should do nothing to make our lives better?

The subsequent chapters are useful in a general sort of way. I list here the chapter titles and a representative quotation from each:

> **2. What Is Parkinson's Disease?:**"Symptoms vary from person to person" (4).

> **3. The Emotional Side of Parkinson's Disease**: "It's important to keep in mind that you are not your disease. You happen to be a person with PD; Your condition is simply a part of who you are" (34).

4. Your Doctor as Partner: "Many of us grew up believing that doctors are somehow magical, that their advice is always right, and that a patient's role is simply to do exactly as the doctor instructs, no questions asked. Times have changed" (37).

5. Drug Treatment for Parkinson's Disease: "Just as people vary widely with PD symptoms, they also vary in their responses to drug treatment" (47).

6. Surgery as Treatment for Parkinson's Disease: "The response to surgery will be only as good as the best response to levodopa" (65).

7. The Importance of Exercise: "Exercise will not stop PD, but it may give you greater strength and independence. It may also improve balance, help you overcome gait problems, strengthen particular muscles, and improve speech and swallowing" (71).

8. Day-to-Day Coping: "Many people, especially those newly diagnosed with PD, resist joining support groups. They prize their independence and don't want to be associated with 'sick people.' This initial resistance usually fades as patients come to grips with their disease" (82).

9. Caring for Caregivers: "Caregiving is difficult—emotionally, spiritually, and physically" (109).

If that sounds new to you, you will probably profit from reading *Understanding Parkinson's Disease*. If you already knew most of it, well, perhaps not.

I should note that in 2017 there appeared a third edition of this book. (See number A30 below.)

A18. *Brain Storms: The Race to Unlock the Mysteries of Parkinson's Disease,* by Jon Palfreman, PhD. New York: Scientific American / Farrar, Straus, and Giroux, 2015. ix + 275 pp.

"There was self-pity. And there was isolation. I didn't reach out to other Parkinson's sufferers. To the contrary, I wanted nothing to do with them. The fragile, bent, trembling figures I observed in neurologists' waiting rooms saddened and angered me. Was this really who I would become?"

B*rain Storms* is a wonderful book. Jon Palfreman has the right credentials for writing a book about Parkinson's: he has a PhD, he is a retired professor in the school of journalism at the University of Oregon, he has had a lot of experience writing and making documentaries about scientific and medical issues, and he has Parkinson's disease. What is most impressive about Jon Palfreman's book is his ability to turn technical, complicated, dry-as-dust science into stories about people. Those stories carry us along three tracks simultaneously.

The first track is the people—from ancient times to the present—who have had or have the disease we now called Parkinson's. The men and women up until the 1960s shook and stumbled their way through a life foreshortened and made miserable by a disease that no one understood and that no doctors could cure. There were not so many of them then as there are now—probably mostly because people tended to die of other causes before they reached the age at which Parkinson's usually showed up. Now, because human life expectancy is longer, there are many more who have the disease. We still shake and stumble, but we shake and stumble less, and we are less miserable. Still no one really understands what causes the disease and still no doctors can cure it. Now, however, neurologists have medicines and surgeries that can help alleviate some of our symptoms for a while. Jon Palfreman keeps the focus on the patients throughout, working in their stories. Some of these people most of us know a little about already—Michael J. Fox and Tom Isaacs come to mind. Others we learn about for the first time, like the dancer Pamela Quinn (see Chapter 4, "Mind Over Matter").

The second track is the neurologists—the physicians, researchers, and scientists—who have struggled to understand and treat this disease. First among these is John Parkinson, the London doctor who two centuries ago, on the basis of six individuals in whom he detected certain features in common, described in "An Essay on the Shaking Palsy" many of the symptoms of the disease that was later named for him. Jon Palfreman tells us about some of the other early scientists: a French researcher and two of his students who through autopsies traced the disease to the substantia nigra, a Russian scientist who discovered the presence of what he called Lewy bodies, two Swedish and Austrian scientists who noticed the absence of dopamine in the brains of patients with Parkinson's, and so on. Jon Palfreman tells us about the later scientists, many of them Americans, who discovered the two most important ways of treating Parkinson's. One of those is carbidopa/levodopa, the medicine that keeps most of us functioning reasonably well. The other is deep brain simulation (DBS), the surgery that implants deep into the brain wires connected to a kind of pacemaker sewn into the chest.

The most interesting story about research is the one about the Israeli woman who, while doing research on Alzheimer's, chanced upon the discovery that a virus known as M13 might be introduced into the nasal passages of mice that had been genetically engineered to develop Alzheimer's disease. She attached to M13 certain man-made antibodies, and found that they got past the blood-brain barrier. She discovered that the virus dissolved the Alzheimer's plaques that were located in the brains of these mice. She then discovered that it also seemed to work on mice with Parkinson's. Later her son, working on an MBA at Harvard, needing to describe a business model of an imaginary company, worked with a classmate to describe a start-up pharmaceutical company based on his mother's discovery. They then decided to borrow enough money to actually set up the company. That company is, last I heard, in the process of seeking FDA approval for trials involving human subjects. If it works as well as they hope it will, it can be used to treat both Alzheimer's and Parkinson's. It has, Jon Palfreman says, the potential to be even more important than carbidopa/levodopa and DBS as treatment for Parkinson's.

The third track is Jon Palfreman himself. *Brain Storms* is in part the story of his learning to deal with his own 2011 diagnosis of Parkinson's disease. He describes honestly his own fears:

I left the hospital in a state of shock. [...] There was secrecy. [...] There was denial. [...] There was self-pity. And there was isolation.

I didn't reach out to other Parkinson's sufferers. To the contrary, I wanted nothing to do with them. The fragile, bent, trembling figures I observed in neurologists' waiting rooms saddened and angered me. Was this really who I would become? (5)

Palfreman decided to read all he could about the disease and to interview neurologists and other scientists about it. He talked with others who had the disease. He gradually learned more and more about the disease and what probably lay ahead for him:

By combining the scientific insights of researchers studying neurochemistry and neurophysiology with the personal experiences of people like Pam, I was beginning to get a deeper understanding of what had befallen me and the challenges I would face down the road. But like other people with Parkinson's disease, I wasn't just interested in understanding what was wrong with me. A part of me hoped for a cure. (62)

That hope was challenged at almost every turn. He discovered, for example, that carbidopa/levodopa and DBS do nothing to stop the disease itself but only treat some of the symptoms, and then only for a while. He discovered that Parkinson's is far more than a "movement disorder." It also affects the digestive system, vision, the voice, and reasoning ability. Jon Palfreman discovered that exercise is vitally important for people with Parkinson's, but also that as their disease progresses, people with Parkinson's are less and less able to do that exercise. He discovered how unlikely it is that the brain cells damaged by Parkinson's can ever be repaired, even if a cure is found. The best he could do was struggle to maintain "a positive attitude, even in the face of scientific setbacks. For as Tom Isaacs once told me, 'If you don't have hope in Parkinson's disease, you don't have anything' " (241).

I learned a lot that I did not know before I read *Brain Storms*. I learned that humans are the only animals that get Parkinson's naturally. I learned about two extended families, one in Contursi, Italy, one in Iowa, in which Parkinson's disease is hereditary. I learned that by 2050 the number of people aged sixty-five and older will triple—meaning that there will be one-and-a-half billion elderly men and women who are of an age where Parkinson's usually presents itself. I learned that by the time we are diagnosed, our brains have already lost about seventy percent of their ability to produce dopamine. I learned that there may be ways to diagnose the disease well before it presents itself through tremor, gait, stiffness, and postural markers, and that the loss of one's sense of smell and the inability to have a bowel movement once a day may well suggest that we have an early stage of Parkinson's. I learned that in drug trials the volunteers taking the placebos often do as well as the volunteers who take the real thing. That suggests that at least some of the time, thinking we are being medicated can be almost as effective as actually being medicated. I learned about the nasty stuff in our brains called alpha-synuclein, which sometimes "goes rogue, forming sticky toxic aggregates that jump from cell to cell inside the brain, killing neurons as they go" (8). I learned how much accident and luck figure in most of the scientific discoveries that have been made about Parkinson's. I learned how important brain autopsies have been in helping scientists understand the nature of Parkinson's. That last made me realize that, just as I have been helped by the autopsied brains of others before me, so I can by donating my brain to science help the many who come after with this disease.

A19. *Carrying the Black Bag: A Neurologist's Bedside Tales*, by Tom Hutton, MD. Lubbock, Texas: Texas Tech University Press, 2015. x + 250.

> "I now realize the angels in the ceiling came to comfort me and keep me from harm."

Dr. Tom Hutton spent most of his professional life as a neurologist in Texas, teaching medical students at Texas Tech and seeing patients, many of whom had Parkinson's. *Carrying the Black Bag* is a bagful of stories. Some are autobiographical, as in the long chapter about how a thumb injury in a high school football practice led to his becoming a doctor rather than a lawyer, and as in the account of the time a sudden snowstorm forced him to midwife his own baby son. Then there was the tale about the man who gave himself small doses of ant-killer poison over an extended period of time hoping to get the VA hospital staff to declare him eligible for disability benefits. In this review I will focus on the chapters that deal with patients with Parkinson's.

In Chapter 8, "The Man Who Played Pinochle with Dogs," Dr. Hutton tells about a seventy-five-year-old country farmer named Sam Woodley who had been diagnosed eight years earlier with Parkinson's. It seems, however, that his medications cause him to have hallucinations in which he is visited by dogs. Furthermore, the dogs have names, they play pinochle with him, and he makes them sandwiches every evening. Sometimes they watch televised football games with him. Dr. Hutton considers changing Sam Woodley's medications, but in the end decides that the imaginary dogs do the lonely old farmer no harm and, indeed, provide him with a healthy sense of companionship. He decides not to change Sam's meds: "For now Sam Woodley would continue to enjoy his extraordinary pinochle parties with 'his dawgs' " (134).

Sam Woodley comes back in Chapter 10, "Pinochle Redux." It is a couple of years later, and Dr. Hutton, having discovered that a mean dog had joined the pinochle pack and frightened Sam, changed the medicines so that the farmer's hallucinations disappeared altogether. Now Sam shows up in the doctor's office bragging—and complaining—about his exciting sex partner, a sixty-year-old Parkinson's patient named Mary Rose. It turns out that Mary Rose is also one of Dr. Hutton's clients. She, in turn, comes in to thank the doctor for giving her that wonderful medicine that makes her feel like a sexy young girl again. Her only complaint is that her boyfriend, Sam Woodley, cannot keep up with her sexual needs: "Sam needs something for, for his manliness. [...] His organ needs tuning, so to speak. [...] Sam's been tailing off on me like a castrated bull" (151). It turns out that one of the medications the good doctor had prescribed for Mary Rose's Parkinson's has had the undesirable effect of making her a compulsive sex addict. He stops the medicine. The tale has a happy ending with Sam Woodley and Mary Rose still enjoying each other's company. They still have sex from time to time, but now having other things to do together, like bowling and enjoying movies, and, yes, playing pinochle.

Chapter 13, "Did Adolph Hitler's Parkinson's Disease Affect the Outcome of World War II?" takes us in a different direction. Dr. Hutton, of course, never met or examined Hitler. But having seen videos of him walking and gesturing, having compared examples over time of his handwriting, and having read various accounts of his behavior, Dr. Hutton feels confident in making a diagnosis-in-absentia. He is reasonably convincing in making the diagnosis of Parkinson's in this case. He is far less convincing in suggesting that if Hitler had not had Parkinson's disease, he would have responded more aggressively to the Allied invasion at Normandy and succeeded in turning back the attack.

In Chapter 14, "Angels in the Ceiling," Dr. Hutton tries to make sense of the strange hallucinations that some Parkinson's patients see as they near death. He gives several examples of these, but focuses particularly on Sarah Simpson, a seventy-seven-year-old retired science teacher who "lay in her recently acquired hospital bed, a place where she fully expected to die" (209). And well she might, since she suffered both from terminal cancer and Parkinson's: "Her Parkinson's disease impaired her ability to move, while the cancer drained her limited energy. She begins to see vague outlines of spirits fading in and out of the ceiling above her bed:

> Sarah's emotional state verged on panic, witnessing the recrudescence of gnarly, bizarre creatures with huge black eyes that stared down at her from the ceiling. She jerked her head from side to side, trying to comprehend this assault that grew from one moment to the next. Anguished and troubled, Sarah felt vulnerable—unable to fight and unable to flee. Fear slaked her diminished stores of fortitude. She observed the strange nonhuman spirits deploy outward from the ceiling's dark corners, as if in formation. They spread like scurrying cockroaches across the ceiling. (210)

Sarah is visited from time to time by a parson named Jerry Brothers. He helps her to take a different view of the spirits she sees in the ceiling. On one of Jerry's last visits to her before she dies, Sarah says:

> "The little people aren't changing anymore. They in fact have developed into the prettiest angels. They make me feel secure. Jerry, I no longer am afraid to die. I now realize the angels on the ceiling came to comfort me and keep me from harm. As you said, they will accompany me on the landing to the distant shore." (217)

Dr. Tom Hutton gives as the subtitle to his book, *A Neurologist's Bedside Tales*. Are these tales true? Well, sort of:

> Real events and patients inspired every story in this volume. The time frames may have been compressed, settings altered, names changed, and at times characters merged due to privacy concerns. I also invented a few minor characters to benefit the storytelling. While the identities and circumstances of patients have been altered to preserve privacy, all the stories are emotionally true. (11)

What does it mean that a tale is "emotionally true" even though the names, times, and settings are falsified, characters are merged and invented? Perhaps it means that Dr. Hutton's bedside tales should be read as fact-based fiction.

A20. *Everything You Need to Know about Parkinson's Disease: The Complete Guide for People with Parkinson's and Their Caregivers* **(revised edition), by Lianna Marie. Copyright 2015 by Lianna Marie. ix + 192 pp.**

> "Even though there is currently no cure for Parkinson's disease, by identifying individual symptoms and determining the right line of treatment, most people with the disease can live enjoyable, fulfilling lives."

Lianna Marie is a freelance writer whose mother Val was diagnosed with Parkinson's around 1990. Lianna Marie learned about Parkinson's disease primarily as her mother's caregiver for a quarter-century. This book has lots of useful information and good advice learned by these two women in the Parkinsonian trenches. It is for the most part simply and clearly written. This is not the book to go to for highly technical medical advice, since the author is not a physician and does not pretend to be. Indeed, she sprinkles her chapters with reminders that Parkinson's is different for everyone who has it, and that readers should always consult their own neurologists about their symptoms and medications. The structure of the book reinforces its lack of depth. Although the book is fewer than 200 pages long, it contains ten parts and sixty-five chapters. There is lots of white space in the book. Each part begins with two pages that are blank except for the title of the part on the first page. Each chapter starts at the top of the page, even though the previous page may have had only a line or two of print. Some chapters are only a half-page long, and rarely does one go over three pages. Complex and nuanced this book is not.

Everything You Need to Know about Parkinson's Disease does, however, have a certain down-home, folksy charm, especially when Lianna Marie talks about her mother's experience with Parkinson's disease. For example, we find these sentences at the end of the short chapter on "How to Increase Mobility":

> My mom [...] tries to get outside everyday to go for a walk. This is to help her keep her mobility for as long as possible (remember the statement: "Move it, or lose it!"). Getting outside also helps prevent

depression, which can often make you lose your motivation to do
any exercise. Sometimes when Mom's mobility isn't that great, she
pushes her wheelchair to help keep her balance and I (or a friend)
walk beside her, there to steady her in case she needs it. Other times
Mom needs no assistance (like when we go shopping—something
Mom absolutely LOVES to do). Parkinson's is funny that way, if
you're really happy or excited about something, sometimes certain
symptoms can seem to disappear. Something else that Mom has
found helpful in increasing her mobility is massage therapy. She
loves this and would go all the time if she could afford it! (155–56)

Before I read *Everything You Need to Know about Parkinson's Disease*, I
had jotted down five questions that I personally wanted the answers to, as
a test to see if the answers were there (I ask similar questions in my review
of Lieberman, *100 Questions*, A13 above): a) What causes Parkinson's? b)
Why has my voice grown weaker and my stutter gotten worse since I was
diagnosed with Parkinson's? c) When my feet "freeze," what can I do to
keep from falling? d) Is it true what I've been told over and over, that you
don't die *of* Parkinson's, but you die *with* it? e) Are we any closer to a cure
for Parkinson's than we were a decade ago?

a) What causes Parkinson's? I was pleased to see that Lianna Marie
has a three-page chapter on "What Causes Parkinson's?" It begins, "As
of this writing, we still don't know what causes Parkinson's" (11). She
mentions the usual possible culprits, like genetics, pesticides, head trauma,
exposure to metals, oxidative stress. She mentions one study that suggested
that people who used either of two pesticides (rotenone and paraquat)
were twenty-five times as likely to get Parkinson's as people who did not.
I don't know if the farmers who farmed near where I grew up in rural
Pennsylvania, used either of those, but I wouldn't be surprised.

**b) Why has my voice grown weaker and my stutter gotten worse
since I was diagnosed with Parkinson's?** Lianna Marie gives no direct
answer to the "why" question, but in her four-page chapter on "Parkinson's
Effect on Speech" she reports that "it is estimated that up to 90% of people
with Parkinson's develop speech and voice disorders during the course of
their disease. Though we don't know exactly what causes these disorders,
researchers think they may be related to the rigidity, slowness, and reduced
range of movement in people with PD." Her only direct mention of
stuttering is this: people with Parkinson's sometimes have "a hurried way of
speaking that sometimes seems like a stutter" (66). Still, I found her advice

to be practical: talk slowly, use short sentences, write down what you want to say, try an amplifier, and so on.

c) When my feet "freeze," what can I do to keep from falling?
Lianna Marie has a page-and-a-half chapter on "How to Prevent 'Freezing'." In that chapter she says nothing about preventing it—a curious gap in a chapter with that title. She does say, however, that "though you may not always be able to prevent freezing, there are some things you can do to help you through it"—like counting, playing music, rocking back and forth, and walking "very carefully backwards or sideways (this works very well for Mom)" (157–58). One of her suggestions is to "try covering your eyes—this can 'trick' your brain and allow you to walk straight ahead with no problems." She does not say what "covering your eyes" means, what we are to cover our eyes with, and how that cover lets us walk straight ahead. It sounds like blindingly dangerous advice. The next chapter (two pages long) is on "How to Prevent Falls." Lianna Marie says that "up to two-thirds of people with Parkinson's experience falls each year" (159). She gives good advice about how to "help prevent falls in your home"—getting rid of small rugs and clutter, installing grab bars in the bathroom, putting handrails on both sides of stairways, and so on. She also offers advice about how to "help prevent frequent falls"—take your meds, wear appropriate footwear (no high heels, or, at home, go barefoot), avoid distractions while walking because "even talking can contribute to falls, as multitasking may be hard for the Parkinson's brain" (160).

d) Is it true what I've been told over and over, that you don't die *of* Parkinson's, but you die *with* it? Lianna Marie's answer is simple and direct: "People do not die from Parkinson's; they die *with* Parkinson's. You may have heard someone say, 'so and so died of Parkinson's,' but this is not true. They may have died from incidents related to the disease, however. […] For example, difficulty swallowing can cause people with Parkinson's to inhale food into their lungs, leading to pneumonia or other lung conditions. Also, loss of balance can lead to falls, which can result in serious injuries or death" (33).

e) Are we any closer to a cure for Parkinson's than we were a decade ago? Lianna Marie has a half-page chapter entitled "Hope for a Cure." Here it is in its entirety:

> Can Parkinson's be cured? Well, we would certainly like to think so. Researchers are still working hard to find a cure, and though they have not found one yet, they have made a lot of progress. There is very real hope that the causes, whether genetic or environmental,

will be figured out, and the exact effects of these causes on how the brain works will be understood. Even though there is currently no cure for Parkinson's disease, by identifying individual symptoms and determining the right line of treatment, most people with the disease can live enjoyable, fulfilling lives. (42)

The answers that Lianna Marie gives to the questions she asks are generally fair and honest, though not profound. I urge readers, however, to be wary of any book about Parkinson's that promises in its title to tell you "Everything You Need to Know about Parkinson's Disease" and to be "The Complete Guide for People with Parkinson's and Their Caregivers." It doesn't and it isn't.

A21. *The New Parkinson's Disease Treatment Book: Partnering with Your Doctor to Get the Most from Your Medications* (second edition), by J. Eric Ahlskog, PhD, MD. New York: Oxford University Press, 2015. x + 525 pp.

> "This book is dedicated to the proposition that PD is not an irreversible sentence to canes, walkers, and disability." […] However, even when disability is in the cards, it often can be forestalled for many years by optimal treatment."

I cannot pretend in a short review to do justice to a 500-plus-page second edition of a book published by an ultra-reputable university press and written by a distinguished physician with thirty years of experience, most of them at the famous Mayo Clinic in Minnesota. Dr. J. Eric Ahlskog is a professor of neurology at the Mayo Medical School and chair of the movement disorders section at the Mayo Clinic.

Dr. Ahlskog describes his book as

> a nuts-and-bolts treatment book addressed to those with PD and their families. It is also meant for the patient's physician, with the intent of making treatment a team approach. After all, physicians, patients,

and families are all on the same team. If patients have a good understanding of not only their disease but also of the appropriate drugs, doses, and the rationale for using these, optimal treatment should be facilitated. (3)

As that statement suggests, Dr. Ahlskog's book is mostly about the various medications available for people who have Parkinson's, how they work, when and in what doses they should be taken, and what side effects they may cause.

Roughly a third of *The New Parkinson's Disease Treatment Book* (Chapters 9–18) deals with the medications typically used in treating the disease. Another third (Chapters 19–29) discusses the long list of "other treatment problems" associated with Parkinson's: sleep issues, dizziness, depression, dementia, hallucinations, delusions, compulsive behavior, drooling, constipation, urinary problems, sexual dysfunction, swelling, vision problems, and so on. The other third takes up various other issues. Chapters 1–8 are about the brain, the changes that Parkinson's brings about in the brain, how to tell if you have Parkinson's, what the prognosis is if you do have it, what it is sometimes mistaken for, what causes Parkinson's disease, and how it typically progresses. Chapters 30–32 take up issues like nutrition, exercise, family, friends, and caregivers. In Chapter 33 Dr. Ahlskog discusses, with undisguised skepticism, surgical options like deep brain stimulation. In Chapter 34 he discusses various experimental options like stem cell transplants. And finally, in Chapter 35, he discusses advocacy and support groups.

If you want to know as much as possible about the medications you are taking or could take, what they can do for you, and what dangers they may involve, and if you are able to follow what are sometimes fairly technical language and explanations, then this would be a good book to have at your bedside. Parkinson's disease is, Dr. Ahlskog says, treatable, especially if we make careful use of the medications currently available:

Parkinson's disease is, indeed, a treatable condition. Medical treatment has increased patients' longevity and allowed most people with PD to remain active and productive for many years. The responses to the available drugs are often striking and occasionally border on the miraculous. PD is among the most treatable of all chronic neurological conditions. (2)

Parkinson's disease is treatable, but the treatments are complex, confusing, and dangerous. Dr. Ahlskog goes on:

> The medical treatment of PD, unfortunately, is not always simple. There are multiple medications available, and these can be used in a variety of ways. The choice of drug, the dose, and the timing often are crucial; therapy must be individualized to meet each person's unique requirements. Also, the distinction between the symptoms of PD and medication side effects is a frequent source of confusion, with potential for ineffective or inappropriate treatment. Sometimes, treatable symptoms are not even recognized as part of PD. The difference between optimal and ineffective therapy may be the difference between a nursing home and independent living. (2)

As that comment on the possibility that we might wind up in a nursing home suggests, Dr. Ahlskog does not want us to forget that there is a lot at stake if we do not take our medications seriously:

> This book us dedicated to the proposition that PD is not an irreversible sentence to canes, walkers, and disability. Admittedly, lives are changed substantially by PD, and for many, the problems will be limiting. However, even when disability is in the cards, it often can be forestalled for many years by optimal treatment. We have medications available to keep people with PD within the mainstream of life; this book addresses how to take full advantage of such treatments. (4)

The New Parkinson's Disease Treatment Book can help you to understand the medications you are taking and recognize the signs when they are not working as they should. If nothing else, it may help you to frame some questions as you prepare for your next visit to your neurologist. Be aware, however, that Dr. Ahlskog's preference for medications rather than nutrition, meditation, exercise, or surgical options is apparent throughout his book, from his subtitle on: *Partnering with Your Doctor to Get the Most from Your Medications.*

A22. *Ten Breakthrough Therapies for Parkinson's Disease*, by Michael S. Okun, MD. Copyright 2015 by Michael S. Okun, published by Books4Patients. x + 145 pp.

> "The first question a patient asks in the office is about his or her symptoms, but the last and most heartfelt is about the research: 'Doc, where is the research going?' "

Chapter 9 of Dr. Okun's earlier book, *Parkinson's Treatments: Ten Secrets to a Happier Life*, is entitled "Always Ask About New Therapies." It begins with this sentence: "The first question a patient asks in the office is about his or her symptoms, but the last and most heartfelt is about the research: 'Doc, where is the research going?' " This second book by Dr. Okun is an extended answer to that question.

In my review of *Parkinson's Treatments: Ten Secrets to a Happier Life* (see A16), I took issue with Dr. Okun's use of the term "secrets" to describe the kind of information he was distributing. That term seemed to invite an accusation of false advertising since it seemed to promise to announce as "secrets" information that most people reading the book would already know. In his new book, *Ten Breakthrough Therapies for Parkinson's Disease*, I have a similar concern: that his term "breakthrough therapies" may mislead potential buyers of the book and cause them to assume that they will find ten breakthrough therapies that will help them now. If they expect that, too many readers will be disappointed.

Dr. Okun defines a breakthrough as a "sudden increase in knowledge, improvement in technique, or fundamental advancement in understanding" (vii). Readers will, after reading this book, wonder just what those ten breakthroughs were. We can easily enough identify two of them—the discovery of carbidopa/levodopa (Chapter 3) and the development of deep brain stimulation (DBS) (Chapter 7), but the other eight are less focused and seem less worthy of being called "breakthroughs." These other eight seem to be large areas where we might hope researchers will in the future make breakthroughs.

In Chapter 1, "Disease Modifying Drugs and Biomarkers," Dr. Okun talks about several drugs and procedures that may someday be used to diagnose or treat the disease. In Chapter 2, "Coffee, Tea, Exercise, Interdisciplinary Teams, and Caregivers," he suggests that caffeine can reduce the risk of getting Parkinson's but does nothing once the disease is in evidence. Exercise helps, but "we have yet to sort out the best types of exercise regimes, the most appropriate frequency of exercise, and the optimal intensity of therapy" (17). He suggests that a patient's family doctor and neurologist should communicate, and that the stresses on caregivers should be carefully monitored.

Chapter 3, "Extended Release/Novel Delivery Systems for Parkinson's Disease Drugs and When to Start Drug Therapy," discusses the discovery a half-century ago of the benefits of L-Dopa as treatment for Parkinson's. That discovery was indeed a true breakthrough at the time, and the various improvements, additives, and delivery alternatives have been used by virtually every living Parkinson's patient.

In Chapter 4, "Marijuana and Synthetic Cannabinoids," Dr. Okun reports that there is little solid evidence that marijuana in any of its various forms helps people with Parkinson's. In Chapter 5, "New Drugs for Hallucinations, Sleep, Constipation, and Dizziness," he reports that several drugs have been in use for these various conditions, but have real or potentially troublesome side effects. For example, using Melatonin for insomnia helps some patients, but for others Melatonin makes it more difficult to sleep. In Chapter 6, "Therapies While Hospitalized and Avoiding Hospitalization," updates Chapter 8 in his previous book. It gives sensible advice about the special problems facing Parkinson's patients who go to the hospital. I had objected in my review of the previous book to the use of the term "treatment" for advice about preparing for a trip to the hospital. I similarly object to his use of the term "breakthrough therapy" for such advice in the new book.

Chapter 7, "Advancing Deep Brain Stimulation Technology, Earlier Intervention, and Dopamine Pumps," one of the chapters that can be said to be about a true breakthrough, discusses the revolutionary practice of implanting electrodes deep into the brain of Parkinson's patients and connecting them to battery packs embedded in the chest. On the horizon are dopamine pumps and ultrasound devices that show some promise of someday letting us live a pill-free life. Chapter 8, "Stem Cells and Stem-Cell Tourism," examines the much-hoped-for and much-hyped-up promise of stem-cell research as a treatment for, or even a cure for, Parkinson's. Dr. Okun explains the many obstacles to success and advises patients never to pay clinics, here or abroad, to give them stem-cell implants. Chapter 9, "Prions and Spreading Proteins, Vaccines, and Growth Factors," presents the idea that Parkinson's disease results from the failure of the brain to rid itself of a bad substance known as alpha-synuclein, which acts like an infection that gradually spreads through the brain. Dr. Okun describes several efforts, some of them promising but none of them yet successful, to attack alpha-synuclein with viruses, vaccines, and gene therapy. The final chapter, "The Drug Development Pipeline," lists some drugs that are now in the process of being tested for safety and effectiveness by the Food and Drug Administration (FDA).

There is much good and useful information in *Ten Breakthrough Therapies for Parkinson's Disease*. The title, however, is misleading. A more accurate title might be *Two Breakthrough Therapies for Parkinson's Disease and Other Therapies that Once Showed or Still Show Promise of Leading to Breakthrough Therapies*.

To his credit, Dr. Okun admits right off that "there has been little progress on an absolute cure" for Parkinson's (1), and he admits that when scientists have found a cure, it will most likely be a cure for only one kind of Parkinson's. In the absence of a realistic anticipation of a cure anytime soon, scientists and medical researchers have devoted their main energies to finding ways to reduce some of the most debilitating symptoms of the disease and to slow down its progression. These are for the most part not really breakthrough therapies, at least not yet, but it is good to know that much good work is going on and that some of those may eventually lead to more breakthrough therapies for Parkinson's disease.

A23. *The Brain's Way of Healing: Remarkable Discoveries and Recoveries from the Frontiers of Neuroplasticity,* by Norman Doidge, MD. New York: Penguin, 2016. xx + 427 pp.

> "This book will show that [...] brain cells being able to constantly communicate electrically with one another, and to form and re-form new connections, moment by moment, is the source of a unique kind of healing."

Most people believe that if you have brain disorders like Alzheimer's, Huntington's, Parkinson's, autism, stroke, attention deficit disorder, and dyslexia, you simply have them. They believe that while you can sometimes lessen or work around some of the symptoms, the damaged brain cannot fix itself. Other parts of the body—the skin, the bones, the liver, and so on—can repair themselves, but the brain you have is the brain you are stuck with. Most scientists have concluded that the brain has evolved into such a sophisticated organ that it is incapable of providing replacement parts for itself.

Norman Doidge, a psychiatrist and a psychoanalyst on the faculty at the University of Toronto, challenges the common notion that a sick brain always remains sick because there is no way for it to heal itself. Dr. Doidge argues in *The Brain's Way of Healing* for the concept of neuroplasticity, the concept that the sick brain is capable of change, improvement, restoration. I quote from his preface:

> It turns out that the brain is not too sophisticated for its own good after all. This book will show that this very sophistication, which involves brain cells being able to constantly communicate electrically with one another, and to form and re-form new connections, moment by moment, is the source of a unique kind of healing. True, in the course of specializing, important reparative abilities, available to other organs, were lost. But some were gained, and they are mostly expressions of the brain's plasticity. (xv)

In this brief review I will deal only with what Dr. Doidge tells us in his long (68-page) chapter on Parkinson's disease. Entitled "A Man Walks Off His Parkinsonian Symptoms," the chapter deals with the claims of John Pepper, the man who wrote the book entitled *Reverse Parkinson's Disease* (2011). Readers may read my review of that book, published below (see number B15). A reminder: John Pepper was an employee of a printing company in Cape Town, South Africa, who had been diagnosed with Parkinson's disease some twenty years before he wrote *Reverse Parkinson's Disease*. In his book he reported that he had discovered that regular, focused, and attentive walking helped his Parkinson's disease, but that carbidopa/levodopa did not. Although he was neither a scientist nor a doctor, he attempted to generalize from his own experience with Parkinson's by urging other people with Parkinson's to follow his example by walking regularly, swiftly, and consciously, and by resisting their neurologist's prescriptions of carbidopa/levodopa.

Near the end of his book John Pepper made the startling revelation that some neurologists had told him that he did not have Parkinson's disease at all, but rather a lesser disease called Parkinsonism—a condition that shared some symptoms with Parkinson's disease, but was quite different. I conclude my review of Pepper's book thus:

We come away from *Reverse Parkinson's Disease* admiring its author's spirit and determination, but unconvinced that his experience is fully relevant to ours. If he never had Parkinson's to begin with, there was nothing to reverse. Until we know for sure, it is best to take this Pepper with a grain of salt.

Dr. Doidge, having recently published to considerable acclaim his first book, *The Brain that Changes Itself* (2007), decided to write a second book in which he related some real-life stories about neuroplasticity. He heard about John Pepper's experiences, read his *Reverse Parkinson's Disease*, then flew to Cape Town for a series of interviews with Pepper, some of them on hiking trails.

Dr. Doidge was amazed at John Pepper's absence of symptoms more than two decades after diagnosis:

> Pepper moves too quickly for a Parkinson's patient. He doesn't appear to have the classic symptoms: no shuffling gait; no visible tremor when he pauses or when he moves; he does not appear especially rigid, and seems able to initiate new movements fairly quickly; he has a good sense of balance. He even swings his arms as he walks. He shows none of the slowed movements that are the hallmarks of Parkinson's. He hasn't been on anti-Parkinson's medication for nine years, since he was sixty-eight years old, yet appears to walk perfectly normally. (33)

How did John Pepper manage, without medications, to rid himself of almost all of the usual symptoms of Parkinson's? He did it, he told Dr. Doidge, by a rigorous walking routine that he had developed for himself. For Dr. Doidge, John Pepper is living evidence of the plasticity of the brain. Neither Dr. Doidge nor John Pepper use the word "cured" for what happened to John Pepper's disease: "his claim was not that he had completely cured himself of the disease; rather, as long as he kept up his walking, he could reverse the main *movement* symptoms of Parkinson's" (37).

Dr. Doidge wonders whether John Pepper had discovered, "through conscious walking, a way of using a different part of his brain to walk" (59). He is aware that "Pepper's critics were arguing that because he was doing better than they expected, he couldn't have had the diagnosis in the first place. They were confusing diagnosis with prognosis and overlooking the fact that he was treating himself very intensively" (72).

Virtually everyone now agrees that people with Parkinson's disease should exercise early, regularly, and intensively. There is no question that it is good for us. It may be wishful thinking, however, to claim on the basis of one patient in a faraway land whose initial diagnosis was questionable that walking causes the brain to create new cells, to heal dead ones, to free us from our reliance on carbidopa/levodopa, or to reverse the downward spiral of Parkinson's disease. We all hope for that kind of progress, but we also hope for more solid evidence for it than we find in either John Pepper's *Reverse Parkinson's Disease* or Norman Doidge's *The Brain's Way of Healing.*

A24. *Everything You Need to Know About Caregiving for Parkinson's Disease,* by Lianna Marie. Copyright 2016 by Lianna Marie. 191 pp.

> "Caregiving isn't for everyone. Though it's tough saying 'no' to your loved one, sometimes it's actually the less selfish, more loving, and more caring thing to do."

In 2015 Lianna Marie (see my review number A20 above) published a book called *Everything You Need to Know about Parkinson's Disease.* Lianna Marie is not a medical doctor. Her knowledge of Parkinson's comes mostly from helping to take care of her mother, who lived with Parkinson's disease, and then also dementia, for a quarter-century. The second book, *Everything You Need to Know about Caregiving for Parkinson's Disease,* is very much a companion to the earlier book. That one had focused on the trials that Parkinson's disease visits on people who have Parkinson's. This new one focuses, rather, on the trials that Parkinson's visits on the person who finds him- or herself responsible for taking care of someone with Parkinson's.

The target audience for this new book is the caregivers themselves, those men and (mostly) women who, by the sudden diagnosis of Parkinson's in someone they love, find themselves suddenly with a companion "diagnosis" as caregiver of an adult with a progressive, incurable, neurological disease. They did not ask for and probably did not want that diagnosis. According to one recent survey, fully half of all caregivers in the U.S. feel that they had no choice about whether they would take on the role as caregiver. It just happened, and there they were, charged with a job for which they had little inclination and no training.

Like the earlier book, which had lots of short, choppy chapters with plenty of white space, this one also has lots of short, choppy chapters with plenty of white space. Most of the information and advice given is helpful, though most of it is pretty-much common sense. Do we really need to be told (in Chapter 1, entitled "Who Cares?") that while some caregivers report that taking care of "their loved one gives them purpose in their lives, [...] many caregivers are overworked, stressed out, or depressed," and that "caregiving can take huge tolls on your health and finances if you're not careful" (3)? More useful is Chapter 3, "Before You Say 'Yes' to Caregiving," where the author gives this sound advice: "Here are three important questions you should answer honestly before you take steps into the caregiving world: 1. Are you physically and emotionally ready? [...] 2. Are you financially ready? [...] 3. Are you legally ready?" That last question has to do with making sure you understand "your loved one's wishes in the end stages of their life. Do they have a plan to pay for their care if needed? Without certain legal documents in place, caring for your loved one can be a lot more difficult than it needs to be" (7–8). The author gives average comparative costs for various kinds of adult care: private room in a nursing home, $90,520/year; assisted living, $42,600/year; home care health aide, $21,840/year (20).

An important feature of this book is its message that it is all right to refuse to be the direct caregiver of someone who is sick:

> Caregiving isn't for everyone. Though it's tough saying "no" to your loved one, sometimes it's actually the less selfish, more loving, and more caring thing to do. Passing the role on to another family member or professional can save you from burning out and may even strengthen your relationship with your loved one if done with love and honesty. (9)

It is interesting that Lianna Marie chose to offer help from a distance to her mother, who suffered for years with Parkinson's. Her mother lived in Canada, while she herself lived 2500 miles away in the U.S. She helped in the early years by offering moral support to her step-father until he himself became too sick to care for his wife, then she arranged for her mother to move to a care facility:

> This helped take the burden off all of us while allowing her to get

the care she needed. I don't consider this to have been us saying 'no' to caregiving, but rather making a choice to care for her in a different way. There is no right or wrong when it comes to the decision of caregiving. Everyone is different and you have to make the choices that are best for you. (9)

Many of the chapters offer advice about specific ways that caregivers can help the person who has Parkinson's: Chapter 27, "Helping with Mobility"; Chapter 28, "Preventing Falls"; Chapter 29, "Managing Freezing Episodes"; Chapter 33, "Help for Drooling and Dry Mouth." Other chapters discuss key decision points: Chapter 43, "When Is It Time to Apply for Disability?"; Chapter 48, "Decisions about Driving: When Is It Time to Take Away the Keys?"; Chapter 50, The Dreaded Nursing Home Decision."

In essence, however, the central focus of this book is how to make life easier for the caregiver who may feel guilty about not doing enough: "Some people [with Parkinson's] have trouble accepting the losses that can accompany Parkinson's, but as rough as it sometimes may be, you need to remember that you're not responsible for your loved one's happiness" (28). "A study from the University of California found that caregivers experiencing extreme stress have been shown to age prematurely. This level of stress can take as much as ten years off a caregiver's life!" (35). "How do you know if you're 'burned out'? If you've reached this state, you will be physically, mentally, and emotionally exhausted. Many caregivers also feel guilty if they spend time on themselves rather than on the loved one" (36–37).

Lianna Marie feels so strongly about guilt that she spends the whole of Chapter 13, "How to Deal with Guilt," on it:

> I wish someone had taught me early on in my caregiving journey about guilt. I wrestled with this emotion for a very long time, not knowing what to do with it or how common it was. Here's a news flash about caregiving: you're going to feel guilty a lot of the time. Guilty for not doing enough. Guilty for not being there enough. Guilty for losing your temper, making wrong decisions, or breaking promises. Guilt was such a part of my life that I felt guilty every time I was having fun and she wasn't. (45)

Lianna Marie has similar chapters on other negative feelings growing out of the stresses of caregiving: Chapter 14, "How to Cope with Loneliness"; Chapter 15, "How to Handle Depression"; Chapter 16, "How to Cope with

Worry of the Unknown"; Chapter 17, "How to Deal with Resentment." Other chapters deal with various other practical issues: Chapter 21, "How Long Will My Caregiving Job Last?"; Chapter 22, "What to Do When No One Will Help"; Chapter 36, "Special Needs of Spousal Caregivers"; Chapter 38, "When Parkinson's Is Keeping You Up All Night"; Chapter 41, "Respite Care"; Chapter 46, "How Do I Find Time for Me?"; Chapter 47, "How to Minimize Caregiver Weight Gain"; Chapter 53, "Grieving While Your Loved One Is Still Alive." These chapters tend mostly to deal with ways to help the caregiver cope with the stresses of caregiving.

In sum, *Everything You Need to Know About Caregiving for Parkinson's Disease* covers a lot of topics, but covers them in very little depth. The focus is more on the needs of caregivers than on how caregivers can help people with Parkinson's. It is written mostly for caregivers, but I would urge people with Parkinson's to read it. Most of us are fully cognizant of the stresses that our disease brings in the lives of those who care for us. This book will remind us of just how serious, demanding, debilitating, and enduring those stresses are. In doing so, it will help us to find ways to give our caregivers some relief, to let them know that we love them, and to assure them that we care about them.

A25. *Goodbye Parkinson's, Hello Life!: The Gyro-Kinetic Method for Eliminating Symptoms and Reclaiming Your Good Health*, by Alex Kerten (with David Brinn). Saline, Michigan: McNaughton and Gunn, 2016. xxi + 205 pp.

> "Once you give the brain and the body the ability to work together and systematically bring them to a new home base, miracles take place."

For most of us, a diagnosis of Parkinson's came in a report from a grim-faced neurologist saying that we have the disease because a deep part of our brain stopped making dopamine. While there was no cure yet, the neurologist told us, the disease moved slowly. With so many scientists searching for a cure, it was only a matter of time until one was found. Meanwhile, there was a growing body of evidence that we could slow down its progression by a regular program of exercise. But the really good news,

the neurologist told us, was that there were a number of effective medicines
with names like rasagiline, ropinirole, and carbidopa/levodopa that did a
wonderful job of managing most of the symptoms of Parkinson's—at least
in the early stages. What we should do was get lots of exercise and take the
medicines that the neurologist prescribed.

Now along comes Alex Kerten, an Israeli physiotherapist who
boldly announces that, yes, exercise is helpful—particularly the specific
exercise program he calls Gyro-Kinetics. He describes Gyro-Kinetics as
a method founded on "the concept of movement, music, and rhythm—
creating motion in the body, which stimulates simultaneous physiological,
biological, and psychological reactions" (xvii). Gyro-Kinetics can,
he assures us in the subtitle of his book, eliminate the symptoms of
Parkinson's.

An important key to understanding his method is what Alex Kerten
calls "listening to your body." His idea is that we get Parkinson's through
one of three causal avenues: 1) genes and heredity, 2) toxins and chemicals,
and 3) behavior: "The overwhelming majority of Parkinson's sufferers
do not fall into either of the first two categories. The most common cause
of Parkinson's disease is chronic behavior that affects and wears out our
nervous system" (17). To effectively fight the disease, Alex Kerten says, we
need to pay close attention to our breathing, to a series of "body forms," to
facial manipulations, to detailed movements and exercises, and to music
and dance. He illustrates these with a series of sixty-odd photographs of
himself in various stances, poses, and movements. To succeed, he says,
we need to commit to learning from him how to correct our behavior and
thus become "Parkinson's warriors"—Alex Kerten's name for the clients
who "come to me to learn how to fight Parkinson's by taking responsibility
through listening and speaking with their body" (9).

What is the role of traditional Parkinson's medicines in the recovery
of a Parkinson's warrior? Alex Kerten's advice is to stay away from those
medicines as much as we can:

> The biggest obstacle to fighting Parkinson's is the medication—the
> complicated cocktails of drugs that can cause side effects we're not
> even aware of. We end up becoming a slave to those side effects
> and their own scenarios as much as we have to our Parkinson's
> symptoms. (56)

While Alex Kerten stops short of insisting that we should refuse all
medications and stay away from the neurologists who prescribe them, he

would have us use his methods first and so reduce the need for so many of those medications:

> Once you give the brain and the body the ability to work together and systematically bring them to a new home base, miracles take place. Now, when you go to the doctor, the medication prescribed based on the symptoms will be a much lower level and can greatly help you instead of being debilitating and leading to harmful side effects. (157)

The evidence that Gyro-Kinetics works is slender and vague. Alex Kerten provides a Foreword by a Dr. Marieta Anca-Herschkovitsch, who visited him at his Gyro-Kinetics facility near Tel Aviv and became convinced that his was the right approach:

> [I] immediately and intuitively realized that it was the correct approach, […] strikingly original and tremendously effective. I suggested to him that we conduct a pilot program to check that effectiveness. We took twelve new clients of his and conducted a general overview of their physical and psychological condition. They then began Alex's program for three months and underwent another checkup. In a subjective manner based on outward appearance, there was unanimous improvement in the subjects' condition. But also objectively, in the scientific scales that I conducted both for their physical and psychological state, there was also significant improvement. (x)

Lots of questions present themselves: How were the twelve clients selected? How long had they been diagnosed? Did they know they were part of an experiment? Was there any sort of control group? What sort of "general overview" was conducted? What sort of "scientific scales" did the investigator employ? How did she define "significant improvement"?

Is the fact that people with Parkinson's make the journey to the Gyro-Kinetics clinic legitimate evidence that Alex Kerten's methods work? Dr. Marieta Anca-Herschkovitsch thinks so:

> His treatment is not inexpensive, yet people make an effort to come to him from around Israel and from around the world. It's not easy for most of them to get there. It must be worth it to them. Because it works and because it makes them feel better. That's the quality

assurance factor—if it wasn't so beneficial, people wouldn't be making the effort to come from all over to get his treatment. (xiii)

Instead of hard research-based evidence that Alex Kerten's system actually works, he gives us testimonials, like the one from a client named Doris Coronel, a fifty-two-year-old woman diagnosed with Parkinson's almost a decade earlier. Impressed with what she had read of the "philosophy behind the Gyro-Kinetics approach, which was 'to help move from being a professional Parkinson's patient to being a healthy person with Parkinson's' " (148), she showed up at his clinic using a walker:

> It's difficult to explain with words the impact that his ten-day, two-and-a-half-to-three-hours-a-day program had on me. The first thing that I regained was my self-confidence; and the first thing I lost, after three days, was my walker. (149).

Talk of miracles and quality assurance and rosy testimonials, however, cannot substitute for hard research, and I leave *Goodbye Parkinson's, Hello Life!* wondering whether Gyro-Kinetics is much more than the delusional ramblings of a narcissist.

Alex Kerten speaks of his "gift": "My gift is my ability to look at people and, based on their behavior, understand if they are balanced in mind and body" (7). If they are not, he shows them how to achieve that balance by becoming a Parkinson's warrior. The true warrior is the one who in a moment of self-awareness says, "Wow, it is so obvious now. I brought Parkinson's upon myself" (7).

But wait. Is it really helpful to tell us folks with Parkinson's that by our own past behavior we have caused the disease? Don't we carry enough guilt in realizing what our disease is doing to our families, without adding to it that we brought it on ourselves? Is it helpful to lead us to believe—or even suspect—that if we do not succeed in "reclaiming our good health" by following Alex Kerten's program, it is because we have not become true Parkinson's warriors? It seems not to occur to the originator of Gyro-Kinetics that the problem may not be our failure as Parkinson's warriors but his failure to understand the nature of Parkinson's disease.

A26. *I Am Rock Steady: Fighting Back against Parkinson's Disease,* by Julie Young. Indianapolis: Dog Ear Publishing, 2016. viii + 149 pp.

> "During a checkup with her neurologist in 2015, the doctor commented that Madeline looked great and there was no need to increase the dosage of her medication."

Rock Steady Boxing is a private exercise corporation based in Indianapolis but with satellite boxing gyms scattered around the United States in places like New Hampshire, Massachusetts, California, Texas, and Florida. There is even one in Italy. The idea is that people with Parkinson's will come to one of the gyms several times a week, strap on their gloves, and fight back against their disease.

Julie Young is a professional writer commissioned by Rock Steady Boxing to write a book about how helpful the program is for people with Parkinson's. She is not a doctor; she is not a science researcher; she does not pretend that she knew much about either boxing or Parkinson's before she accepted the commission.

To gather information for *I Am Rock Steady*, Julie Young interviewed the founder of Rock Steady Boxing, members of the staff, and ten of the company's satisfied clients. The core of the book is the ten chapters on the satisfied clients. These chapters follow a predictable formula: what the clients did before being diagnosed with Parkinson's, their distress at receiving the diagnosis, how they learned about Rock Steady Boxing, and how the program has helped them.

Typical is Chapter 3, focused on the experience of Madeline O'Mara of Amherst, New Hampshire. After graduating from college she got a good job as an electrical engineer. After twenty years with the company she was laid off and took a new job as a software engineer with a computer company. After a couple of years there, she began to notice tremors in her right hand and leg. Her family doctor suggested that she see a neurologist, who after examining her told her she had Parkinson's. She then began what she called "the unceasing and ever-changing dance with drugs" (36). The drugs helped with her tremors but made her sleepy and led to a couple of automobile accidents. She eventually decided to quit that job and changed neurologists. With this new one she began a "search for the elusive Holy Grail of medicinal concoctions" (37). Her new doctor told her that exercise was vital for people with Parkinson's.

   She knew she had to do something: "Madeline couldn't rise from a chair without using her arms, her gait was slow and unsteady, and she fell daily because her balance was poor" (39). She heard about Rock Steady Boxing from a medical technologist when she went for her annual mammogram: "the tech told her she had a colleague whose husband was also a Parkinson's patient. The tech said the husband has found boxing to be extremely helpful both physically and from a therapeutic standpoint. Madeline was intrigued to hear more" (40). She eventually found a Rock Steady Boxing class not far from where she lived and signed up in March 2014. It was rough going at first, but:

> On her first-year anniversary in the Rock Steady Boxing program, there was no question that Madeline was stronger and had better range of motion, better motivation, and better stamina. When she lost her balance in the past, she would fall. Thanks to the program, she now has the ability to catch herself. On those occasions when she does fall, she knows how to fall correctly in order to avoid injury. In addition to the physical benefit, Madeline says the program gives her a wealth of intangibles, such as camaraderie, support, and a family unit that she never could have imagined. During a checkup with her neurologist in 2015, the doctor commented that Madeline looked great and there was no need to increase the dosage of her medication. (42)

"Thanks to Rock Steady Boxing," Madeline says in the last line of the chapter, "I am physically and mentally stronger than before" (43).

   Perhaps so, but there is in the ten chapters no mention of anyone who had a bad experience, no mention of anyone who got hurt, no mention of clients who left the program, no mention of a control group, no mention of pre- or post-tests designed to measure improvement objectively. All we find is one testimonial after another of people selected because they liked the Rock Steady Boxing program.

   A line on the front cover of the book identifies it as "Inspirational stories about the courageous boxers of Rock Steady Boxing as told to Julie Young." Read *I Am Rock Steady* if you want to, but read it knowing that you are reading not an objective research report but advertising copy designed primarily to inspire you to sign up for a class.

A27. *On My Own,* by Diane Rehm. New York: Alfred A. Knopf, 2016. 162 pp.

> "I'm reaching back in time, reaching back before John grew weak, when he was still able to lift the twenty-five-pound bird from the oven."

Diane Rehm, the anchor of National Public Radio's *The Diane Rehm Show*, was married for fifty-four years to John Rehm. In June 2014, at age eighty-three, John decided to end a life made impossible by Parkinson's. He could no longer clean, feed, or dress himself, move without assistance, do any kind of meaningful work, or enjoy much of anything about his daily existence. He knew that no cure for Parkinson's could come in time to help him. He knew that his life could grow only more impossible, that he would grow only more dependent on others, that his daily care would grow only more expensive in the weeks and months ahead. After discussing his decision with his wife, his son, and his daughter, he asked his doctor to give him lethal drugs. His doctor refused because the laws in the state of Maryland, which had not provided any meaningful death-with-dignity options, forbade physician-assisted death. The doctor said he could keep John comfortable if he decided to end his own life by refusing food, water, and medicines. John Rehm acted on that information, and ten days later, he died.

John's nickname was Scoop. Diane starts her book with Scoop's death. It was a death that made her feel a complex array of conflicting emotions: relief, sadness, loneliness, freedom, fear, frustration, nostalgia, guilt, love, resentment, anger. These emotions all gain full expression in her book, which can be read as a kind of grief diary. It is a realistic book that many who have Parkinson's or who love someone with Parkinson's will want to read. Some may find it depressing to learn in so much honest detail about what this disease can do to people, and to the families of people, with the disease. It is not always a pretty story, but it is a lovely one.

In her short chapter entitled "November 23, 2014," Diane addresses some questions to her husband on what would have been his eighty-fourth birthday if he had not died six months earlier:

> How are you? Has the journey been what you'd hoped it might be? Is that new world as peaceful and as filled with light as we here on earth want to imagine? Can you "feel"? Are you strong? Does

it matter? Can you see me? Can you understand how I have been
longing to speak with you? (106)

Scoop, of course, cannot answer his widow's questions directly, but here
is an imagined response that he might have given:

My Dearest Diane:
   I will not answer all of those questions. You'll know the answers
soon enough, when you make the journey. But I have read your
book and I want to thank you for writing so eloquently about our
romantic but sometimes lonely marriage, and your own life pre-me,
with-me, and post-me. I appreciate your willingness to share with
the world so much about the shifting joys and distresses of our long-
running marriage. I especially appreciate your public call for laws
that provide for greater self-determination in dealing with terminal
illnesses. The world generally lets us live the lives we want to live,
marry the people we want to marry, have the children as we want
to have, divorce when we want to divorce, retire when we want
to retire. We get to make all of those huge life-altering decisions
on our own. Why does the world refuse to let us exit life when the
time comes? Why does the world insist that we live on well past the
time when we are capable of doing anything meaningful, learning
anything worth knowing?
   I want to talk about three subjects you raise in your book:
silence, guilt, and erasure.
   Silence. You speak about my long silences, about my punishing
you by shutting you out of my life. I did that and I am sorry. Much
of that silence was the result of a damaged ego brought on by your
wonderful success. You say that I was your teacher, the man who
encouraged you, who provided the college education you never
had. Do you remember My Fair Lady, that musical we saw many
years ago? You were Eliza Doolittle to my Henry Higgins. Professor
Higgins surely felt great pride in seeing his fair lady succeed in
her brave new world, but he must also have felt a measure of
envious amazement as Eliza outgrew him. As your radio career
took off and my legal business declined, as your salary went up and
mine went down, I felt both proud of your accomplishments and
resentful of them. I would not have wanted you to fail, but it stung
me to have your big successes make my little successes look like
failures. When my Parkinson's diagnosis came shortly after the

automobile accidents that forced me to give up driving, I began to feel even more useless and even more dependent on you for almost everything. All that shut me up. Forgive me, please.

Guilt. You say in your book that you have at times felt guilty about our decision that I should move to an assisted living facility away from home. Please don't feel guilty. No one wants to have to move to such a place, but I preferred that to having you quit the work you loved so you could stay home and take care of me. I knew how much your NPR show meant to you and to your millions of listeners world-wide. I knew how much we both depended on your income. Can you understand that the very last thing people with Parkinson's want is to be a burden to those we love? We want to do all we can to pull our own weight. When we can no longer do that, and when we must reluctantly let others do for us what we used to do for them, it is far less ourselves we feel sorry for than them. It is easier for us to see ourselves being sucked down by our disease than to see our disease suck down others. That makes us feel guilty. But hey! Let's both agree to stop feeling guilty. Deal?

Erasure. In the chapter that you wrote on what would have been my eighty-fourth birthday, you say that you work hard to remember me as I used to be.

> I'm reaching back in time, reaching back to before John grew weak, when he was still able to lift the twenty-five-pound bird from the oven. In fact many of my memories of him have begun to shift from after he became ill to before. I want to remember him as he was when he was younger and stronger, not necessarily in his twenties or thirties but in his forties and fifties, before any back problems or operations, before any slowing down or shuffling. I want to remember him as he swung a pickax to break up the driveway in front of our house on Worthington Drive. I want to see him as he hauled a wheelbarrow full of tree trimmings at the farm or when he lifted large pieces of rock to repair the stone wall. I want to feel his arms as he carried me up the stairs at our first dwelling in Georgetown. (108)

I understand why you want to remember me as I once was rather than as I became, but I ask you please not to erase the man that I became. I was once stronger, louder, and manlier, but the true measure of my manhood came later, after I was diagnosed. I am not proud of the way I handled all that, but my Parkinson's years were an important part of me and of us. I urge you not to erase them by leapfrogging back to my glory days. My final years were my glory days.

Thank you. I love you.

Scoop

A28. *Optimal Health with Parkinson's Disease: A Guide to Integrating Lifestyle, Alternative, and Conventional Medicine*, by **Monique L. Giroux, MD. New York: Demos Medical Publishing, 2016. xxi + 295 pp.**

> "This book is written to help you live and thrive. It is intended to help you move beyond a reductionist and traditional approach defined by symptoms to an integrative or holistic approach."

After beginning her medical practice in the greater Seattle area, Dr. Monique Giroux moved her practice, which she calls the Movement and Neuroperformance Center, to Colorado. Her approach, in her practice and in her book, is to encourage people with Parkinson's to take a wide view of their health: "You are not your disease. But you are living with your disease. Living your best, then, means a focus that extends beyond the treatment of symptoms. [...] This book is written to help you live and thrive. It is intended to help you move beyond a reductionist and traditional approach defined by symptoms to an integrative or holistic approach" (xii).

Optimal Health with Parkinson's Disease is improved by several features. Interspersed throughout are two kinds of boxed asides. First are the "Clinical Pearls" that give special information on specific issues like how to talk to your neurologist about integrative therapies (47–48). Then there are the boxed "Interviews with the Experts" about specific questions. The interview with Terry Ellis of Boston University, for example, shows how physical therapists and personal trainers can help people with Parkinson's (77–80). Another helpful feature is the list of references at the end of each chapter to guide readers to articles on specific studies relating to information given in that chapter.

After a general overview of Parkinson's disease in Part I—its causes, its medical and surgical therapies, and the usefulness of a more integrative approach—Dr. Giroux moves in Part II to a wide-ranging discussion of general health. She warns against thinking of Parkinson's disease as an isolated phenomenon. She warns against thinking that all we have to do is treat the Parkinson's, and all will be well. She warns against thinking that if we did not have Parkinson's, we would be healthy, vigorous, and cheerful, and would live forever. No, no. The average age at diagnosis is just under sixty. That is about the age when the aging process becomes evident in most people. Our problem, then, is not merely that we have Parkinson's, but also that we are growing older. She also talks about "lifestyle medicine"— including weight management, intake of alcohol, exercise, nutrition, stress management, mindfulness, and creativity.

The thing I like best about *Optimal Health with Parkinson's Disease* is its broad scope. It focuses, to be sure, on the needs of people with Parkinson's, but it surrounds those needs with a wealth of information that is useful for anyone seeking optimal health. We need to consider the health needs of the whole person, not just that part of the person that has a particular movement disorder. Dr. Giroux says that taking good care of our general health can help to ward off or postpone the start not only of Parkinson's, but also of other kinds of health problems like heart disease, stroke, and diabetes. She tells us, for example, that "in a large study analyzing current and prior exercise habits of 48,574 men and 77,254 women, exercise reduced the risk of developing PD. The effect was stronger in men than women and notable for both current exercise regimes and exercise in early adulthood" (69).

One if the most engaging features this book is its wide inclusiveness. For Dr. Giroux, it is not enough to treat Parkinson's by prescribing carbidopa/levodopa and deep brain stimulation, though those are often a necessary part of the treatment. Part III describes a large number of what she calls integrative therapies: "biological therapies" (including vitamins and minerals, antioxidants, glutathione, turmeric, coenzyme Q10, foods that are especially good for people with Parkinson's, probiotics or helpful bacteria, botanicals like marijuana and St. John's Wort); "body therapies" (including chiropractic manipulations, the Feldenkrais method, massage, music, dance, tai chi, qigong, and yoga); "mind-body therapies" (including biofeedback, breathwork, hypnosis, meditation, and mindfulness); "energy and sensory medicines" (including acupuncture, aromatherapy, therapeutic touch, light therapy, magnet therapy, Reiki, and vibration therapy); "community, spirituality, expressive, and experiential healing" (including animal therapy, journaling, music and art therapy, nature or ecotherapy, spiritual healing and prayer, support groups, volunteerism); and "whole systems approaches" (including Ayurvedic medicine, homeopathic medicines, and traditional Chinese medicine).

In Part IV Dr. Giroux talks in some detail about specific strategies that have proven useful in treating the motor symptoms of Parkinson's— symptoms like bradykinesia, rigidity, dyskinesia, tremor, problems with walking, balance, and freezing of gait. She gives a disappointingly short half-page chat showing some possible integrative approaches to these symptoms, then moves on to ways of treating non-motor symptoms like anxiety, apathy, cognitive decline, constipation, urinary problems, depression, fatigue, insomnia, nausea, and restless legs. For many readers Part IV will be of greatest interest because it offers possible treatments for specific symptoms.

Then, in Part V, Dr. Giroux suggests strategies for personalizing your care by making a plan, assembling what she calls an "integrative team," and gathering together health and life style tools. Some readers may find themselves to be mildly annoyed by the implication in Part V that people with Parkinson may not be sufficiently motivated to do the work necessary to take charge of their own therapy. She suggests that we ask ourselves questions like these:

> How motivated am I to change? [...] Is my interest in making healthy change strong or am I following the desires of others? [...] Do I believe these changes would make a difference? [...] What are a few small steps I can take to move toward my goal? [...] How will I keep up with my goal? (256)

It may well be that the reason we sometimes fail to make much headway against the ravages of Parkinson's is that we are not sufficiently motivated. But let's not forget that Parkinson's has all the aces and one-eyed jacks. With motivation, smarts, experience, luck, careful playing of the hands we are dealt, and an occasional bluff, we can win a few hands, but Parkinson's holds all the winning cards.

A29. *Road to Recovery from Parkinson's Disease,* by Robert Rodgers, PhD. Copyright Parkinson's Recovery, 2017. 375 pp.

> "My suggestion is quite simple. Give your body a chance to heal itself. Yes, it takes time. Yes, it takes patience. The body knows how to heal itself."

Robert Rodgers has a PhD degree. He does not tell us the subject of his doctorate, but he lets us knows right off that it is not in medicine: "I am not a medical doctor. I am not qualified to address issues you may be having with medications" (21). Having said that, he proceeds to tell us a few pages later that these medicines are not good for us. It is obvious from start to finish that Robert Rodgers has a deep, almost visceral, distrust of the traditional Western medicines that most neurologists prescribe for their Parkinson's patients. Indeed, he is convinced that traditional Western medicines killed his mother:

> Medications do not address the cause of the systems. They suppress symptoms temporarily. This is why the medications have to be taken day in and day out the rest of your life, often in higher and higher doses to maintain the same result. [...] My mother was diagnosed with Parkinson's. She wound up taking an array of ten different medications—some were prescribed to treat her Parkinson's symptoms and others to treat a variety of other problems. I am convinced she died from taking too many prescribed medications at the same time. (42)

One of the traditional truisms of Parkinson's disease is that it is "degenerative" and "progressive"—that is, that the characteristic symptoms of the disease will over time get worse and worse. These are not facts, according to Robert Rodgers, but beliefs, and "these beliefs are blatantly false" (20). He draws a curious distinction between the terms "recovery" and "cure." People with Parkinson's, he insists, can with effort recover from the disease—or at least put themselves on the "road to recovery"—but he holds out no hope for a cure. One of the distinctions he makes between the two terms is that recovery is something you do for yourself now, while a cure is something you wait for someone else to do for you in the future.

Another is that recovery is a process that will occupy you for the rest of your life, while a cure is a pill or an operation that will supposedly fix you once and for all: "By recovery I do not mean to suggest that the condition is 'cured' but that there is sustained relief from the symptoms of Parkinson's" (24). A more accurate title for this book, then, might be *Road to Sustained Relief from the Symptoms of Parkinson's Disease*.

The road to this sustained relief is shifting and complex, but it is anchored in what Robert Rodgers calls "natural therapies":

> I do not have Parkinson's myself. If I did, I would pursue a wide variety of diagnostic protocols to assess the causes and pursue natural therapies to address these causes. The natural therapies that offer the promise of help depending on the cause are many: Biophoton therapy, BioAcoustic therapy, quantum healing, bioenergetics assessments, NES Health, homeopathy, craniosacral therapy, acupressure, herbs, essential oils, Bach Flower essences, aromatherapy, light therapy, hypnotherapy, voice profiling, Emotional Freedom Technique, energy healing, Healing Touch, Reiki, psychics—and this is a short list!
>
> I would also elect to eat live organic food that my body needs to recover and exercise regularly. I believe in my heart that recovery from any disease is possible and have set my intention to document story after story of recovery from the symptoms of Parkinson's. I thus document the various ways to diagnose the causes and the therapies and treatments that offer the possibility of relief. (20)

The stories that he "documents" are mostly drawn from his 200-plus radio interviews on his show called *Parkinson's Recovery Radio*. His guests on the show have been varied:

> Some guests have the symptoms of Parkinson's and discuss the therapies they have found that reverse them. Other guests are health care practitioners, including medical doctors, naturopaths, homeopaths, researchers, neural feedback practitioners, physical therapists, psychologists, herbalists, aroma therapists, neuro-linguistic programming (NLP) therapists, hypnotherapists, music therapists, energy healers—and this is only a partial list! (27)

I cannot here review the many radio interviews that Robert Rodgers refers to in his book. For those interested in following them up, he gives the URL of the archive and the dates of the various interviews. I want, rather, to glance at a few of the generalizations that he makes as a result of his research. For example, he reports that two factors determine which individuals will succeed in their quest for recovery: "First, if you believe in your heart that you can recover, you will recover." (38). That way of putting it gets him off the hook. If what he recommends fails, then the failure is yours, not his, because you did not really "in your heart," believe it would help. He goes on:

> Second, people who see a relief of symptoms know that their healing comes from a place deep inside themselves. That is to say, healing comes from within, not without. They take full charge of their program of recovery. People who experience a gradual deterioration in their health tend to hold the belief that their healing must inevitably come from a source outside themselves. They want to be fixed by medicines or surgeries. (38)

Again, if his suggestions fail, it is your own fault because you believe that you can be helped only by traditional "outside" medical practices.

Robert Rodgers speaks of the human body as if it were its own doctor. He says over and over in his book that we must learn to "listen" to our bodies (39, 69, 75–78, etc.). If we do, it will let us help it heal itself:

> My suggestion is quite simple. Give your body a chance to heal itself. Yes, it takes time. Yes, it takes patience. The body knows how to heal itself. I am acknowledging here what people have known for thousands of years. We simply forgot the truth of who we really are. It is high time to reclaim the wisdom of our ancestors. (53)

Much good information and advice can be found in *Road to Recovery*. The author has helpful things to say about some of the known causes of Parkinson's disease (pesticides and herbicides), about how important it is for people with the disease to avoid wheat, dairy, and sugar, to eat organically-grown foods, and to exercise every day. He says some flattering things about people with Parkinson's: that they are more "successful" and "creative" than people who do not have the disease.

Robert Rodgers tells us early in his book that his "research findings" suggest that "as many as three-fourths of persons diagnosed with Parkinson's disease actually have something else wrong" (20). He does not discuss the nature or scope of that research, and he does not tell us how to verify whether or not we really have the disease. Furthermore, he appears not to understand the dual problem that his research, if it is reliable, raises. If, indeed, three out of four of us who have been diagnosed with Parkinson's have actually been misdiagnosed, then his advice about how to recover from the disease is not relevant to most of his readers. More serious is the implication that if three out of four people with the diagnosis do not have the disease after all, then many of the patients that he interviewed on his radio show probably did not have the disease to begin with, so their "recovery" from it is meaningless.

In the end, according to Robert Rogers, the important thing is what we believe about Parkinson's disease. If we think we have "a disease which is predestined to get worse over time, this is precisely what will happen" (68). Alternatively, "if we believe that we can heal from disease, we will heal" (68). He makes it sound so simple. Actually, that does sound pretty simple. Robert Rodgers makes similar points in his 2012 book, *Pioneers of Recovery* (see number A14 above).

A30. *Understanding Parkinson's Disease: A Self-Help Guide* (third edition), by Steven H. Schechter, MD, and David L. Cram, MD. Omaha, Nebraska: Addicus Books, 2017. xii + 152 pp.

This third edition, now listing Dr. Schechter as the lead author, Dr. Cram second, and Dr. Gao not as all, is very similar to the second edition (see number A17 above). It has essentially the same nine-chapter structure. It adds a number of illustrations, updates the discussion of deep brain stimulation, and mentions new delivery systems for carbidopa/levodopa, Specifically, it mentions Rytary (a time-release pill) and Duodopa (a pump system that meters the medicine directly into the small intestine). Most of the text in the second edition is repeated verbatim in the third, including all of the bits that I quoted in my review of the second edition.

Shelf B: Nonfiction Books about Parkinson's by People with Parkinson's

B1. *The Parkinson's Handbook,* **by Dwight C. McGoon, MD. New York: W. W. Norton, 1990. 175 pp.**

> "Don't be too proud to accept help, yet avoid premature invalidism. Celebrate each victory; praise yourself and your care partner at every opportunity."

Dwight C. McGoon was a successful surgeon at the Mayo Clinic when Parkinson's struck, forcing him to give up surgery. So far as I know, he was the first doctor with Parkinson's to write a book about the disease. It is, as we might expect, sometimes a bit technical in its explanations. Dr. McGoon uses terms like axon, dendrite, motor pathway, synaptic vesicle, substantia nigra, striatum, and so on. He defines such terms as he goes. He is aware that lay readers will have trouble following his explanations, and he finds ways of letting us know that it is all right not to understand it all: "Please don't worry if you're not fully grasping all of this information, which may be of interest to some readers but is by no means essential" (27).

One of the most attractive features of *The Parkinson's Handbook* is the author's no-nonsense bluntness. Are the medicines our neurologists prescribe curative?

> Let us be clear about one fact. At present, there is no such thing as a cure for Parkinson's disease. Certain drugs modify and ease the

symptoms and signs of the disease. But despite the ingenuity with which they are devised, each of them, in whatever combination or dosage schedule, falls short of restoring our normal state. All known treatments are purely palliative. They "ease without curing." (47–48)

Is there a cure in the works?

No current treatment attacks the root cause of the problem, because the root cause is unknown. Present treatments are only attempts to patch up some of the disturbing effects of a causative agent or process. History discloses abundant evidence that until the true cause of a disease is understood, preventive or curative treatment will remain elusive. (57)

Will we be a burden to those whose fate it is to take care of us?

We must be forever aware that we Parkinson's patients do, indeed, impose a burden on those who care for us. Our loved ones may not, because of their deep-felt concern for us, regard our care as a burden, but in fact it is certainly that. We must, early on, resolve to remain as self-sufficient as possible. And it would be extremely wise for us to decide in advance what course of action to adopt when self-sufficiency becomes impossible. (74)

Dr. McGoon comes close to apologizing for the fact that his book is "highly personal, being extensively based on my own experiences with Parkinson's" (9); "Because I myself have the disease, I inevitably introduce many personal anecdotes and examples" (21). Surely, however, no apologies are necessary. Dr. McGoon's personal experiences are the best thing about the book. One of my own favorite bits is his account of his evening walks. Is there any of us who does not resonate with his desire to be invisible when he goes out?

Late evening seemed the ideal time—just after dark—since my telltale stooped posture and faltering steps might then be less apparent to any chance passersby. Furthermore, the slight physical fatigue induced by the pre-bedtime exercise might lead to a better night's sleep. All through the day, I looked forward to that stroll— to the enjoyment of being out in various weather conditions; to the thrill of being able to walk fairly normally (even though the immediate effects of that day's medications had by then essentially dissipated); to the vicarious pleasure of imagining the family doings in those well-groomed homes that I passed; to the satisfaction of greeting, on clear evenings, the few planets and constellations familiar to me. (69)

Although he says that he writes about his own experiences and insists that people with Parkinson's are all unique, in fact, a great deal of what he writes about will sound familiar to many of us: difficulties in dressing ourselves, difficulties reading books held in shaking hands; difficulties writing, typing, and speaking; difficulties shifting position in bed; difficulties traveling; difficulties with constipation, urination, and sexual issues; difficulties with walking, freezing, and falling. I particularly appreciated reading what Dr. McGoon says about the frustrations of freezing:

There I stood, once again, wanting to go down to the basement, but frozen to a spot in the kitchen about two and a half feet from the basement stairway—frustrated to my very core. I know that if I could just get that first foot over onto the top stair, the rest of the way down would be easy. Still, my feet wouldn't budge. Sometimes I had the urge to cry or to throw something through a window. Or why not just abandon all caution and force myself to lean forward until, off balance, I could plunge head-first down that forbidding stairway, and hope for the best? (103–04)

I could have written those lines this afternoon. Twice.

Dr. McGoon closes his book with an important chapter on what he calls "attitude." He starts with a statement of fact: "Like it or not, we who are afflicted with Parkinson's disease face an inescapable challenge. Our pressing concern is whether we can react to its onslaughts with steadfast optimism and hope or must give in to despondency and despair" (133). Not surprisingly, he opts for optimism and hope. He argues that people with Parkinson's are actually better off than most people. The disease is slow-moving, giving us more time after diagnosis to enjoy life and to grow spiritually. The disease is relatively painless. It comes with no guilt attached, since we did nothing knowingly to bring the disease on. Its effects are more physical than mental, leaving our ability to think, understand, and learn mostly intact. Besides, there are medicines that can help us manage some aspects of the disease. And though Parkinson's disease is incurable, it is rarely the actual cause of death. Even if it were, it is not as if not having Parkinson's would let us escape the inevitability of death. Death will come; we should not forget that there are worse diseases to die of or with than Parkinson's.

Dr. McGoon gives some predictable closing advice in the form of "resolutions." For example: "Maintain motivation and enthusiasm for life. Exercise intelligent, though realistic, courage. Fight back and try to overcome. Search for new solutions and ways to resist. Practice caution and carefulness." Yes, yes. Decent enough advice for anyone with a problem. Only the last two of his "resolutions" seem specific to people with Parkinson's: "Don't be too proud to accept help, yet avoid premature invalidism. Celebrate each victory; praise yourself and your care partner at every opportunity" (143).

The Parkinson's Handbook is dated—it does not mention deep brain stimulation, for example—but is still useful, especially for what it reveals about its author's own remarkable attitude toward his disease, our disease. Dr. McGoon died in 1999, at age 73. According to his obituary, he died "from complications of Parkinson's disease."

B2. *Saving Milly: Love, Politics, and Parkinson's Disease*, by Morton Kondracke. New York: Ballantine, 2001. xxi + 229 pp.

> "I can't stand to live this way anymore. I'd rather die."

Many books have been written by people with Parkinson's. Those books are typically written by men and women who want to tell about the early stages of the disease. They tell about their first uncertain symptoms—usually a slight tremor, or increasingly illegible handwriting, or a dragging left foot, or a right arm that doesn't swing when they walk. Then they tell about their visit to their family doctor, who scratches his head and refers them to a neurologist. The neurologist gives them a series of physical tests: "Walk down the hall and back; good; touch your right thumb to your right index finger and then to the other fingers on your right hand; good; can you do it faster?; good; now do that with your left hand; good; can you please take off your shoes so I can see if the soles are equally worn?; good; thanks; now put them on again so I can give you a quick balance test."

When all that is done, the neurologist says, "Well, something's going on, but I'd like you to go to the lab for an MRI to rule out the possibility of a clot or a brain tumor; then come back and we'll see what we find out."

Then the writers of these books tell about the diagnosis, which often sounds something like this: "I think you have Parkinson's, but it's a slow-moving disease; it is easily treated with medications and even brain surgery; Parkinson's won't kill you; there is no cure yet, but a lot of resources are being devoted worldwide to finding one, which researchers are likely to find in five or ten years." The writers of these books tell about the importance of having a positive attitude, of exercising, of going to support groups, of maintaining a sense of humor, of showing gratitude and sympathy for your caregiver, and so on.

The writers of these mellow books end their stories well before the going gets really rough. They do so for two reasons. First, they want to end their books on a positive note, not a downer. Second, by the time their Parkinson's disease reaches the later stages, they will probably, because of the limitations imposed by the disease, have become unable to think, speak, or write clearly about what is going on with them.

Saving Milly is not that kind of book. Unlike most books about the experiences of people with Parkinson's, this one was written by the spouse of a person with Parkinson's. And not just any spouse. Morton Kondracke is a well-known Washington, DC, journalist who casually drops the names of people he has spoken with about the politics of funding for research into Parkinson's: Michael J. Fox, Bill and Hillary Clinton, George W. Bush, John McCain, and others. He describes the earliest signs of the disease in his wife Milly, and he carries the story not just through the relatively easy early mellow stages, but almost to the bitter end. Indeed, in a sense he begins his story at the bitter end:

> Parkinson's disease has kidnapped my wife. It is in the process of killing her. I hug and kiss what is left of her, hang photographs of the old, strong Milly throughout the house, and talk to her. We hold hands. We make love. But she is not who she was. She cannot walk, and now she can barely speak. She is being carried into an abyss, and I am helpless to rescue her. [...] Virtually unable to swallow, Milly is now being sustained through a feeding tube. She can stay alive, but she is likely to be a prisoner in her body, able to understand but unable to communicate. (xvii, xix)

The first two chapters of *Saving Milly* are about Millicent Martinez's birth and growing up in Chicago, about her meeting and ultimate marrying Morton Kondracke, and about their stormy marriage and their two daughters. The third chapter deals with the "invasion" of Parkinson's into the forty-eight-year-old Milly's life, about Milly's worst-case fears —"You'll have to take me to the bathroom. You'll have to feed me" (55)— and about her desperate attempts to try various medical, spiritual, and alternative strategies to stop or slow the progression of the disease. The fourth chapter is about two surgical procedures Milly tries, pallidotomy and deep-brain stimulation, neither of which do her any real good.

The fifth chapter focuses on the dramatically altered roles that Milly and Morton Kondracke are forced into by Milly's worsening condition. Milly had always been the domestic leader, the independent one, the "I-can-do-it" partner, allowing Morton to go about building his career as a Washington correspondent to the *Chicago Sun-Times* and as a long-term panelist on *The McLaughlin Group*. Now, however, as Milly continues to fall (literally and repeatedly) into dependency, Morton finds that he has to take charge of his family and take care of his wife. As her motor skills deteriorate, he becomes the pusher of her wheelchair, the one who hires women to look after her when he has to be at work. He has to try to cheer her up—usually not very successfully or for very long—when she falls into despair and demands, for example, to know why God is punishing her:

> The best I can say to Milly is that I do not think God is punishing her for anything or that God inflicted Parkinson's upon her. I tell her that, as they say, "shit happens"—and for some reason God allows it to happen. He is also available, however, to provide comfort and instill courage. This works for me, but it does not work for her. (115)

In the sixth and seventh chapters, Morton Kondracke describes his decision to become a political activist as he tries to figure out why research for some diseases—like HIV/AIDS and breast cancer—are richly funded with federal dollars, while Parkinson's gets much less federal research support. Once he figures it out he becomes a serious advocate for Parkinson's research. He writes an impassioned column about Parkinson's victim Morris Udall, by then totally bedridden and on feeding tubes. Morton Kondracke makes direct appeals to prominent politicians. He asks for votes, support, dollars.

In the last chapter, both Morton and Milly Kondracke realize that no research dollars or medical breakthroughs will save Milly. She has become almost as bad off as Mo Udall had been at the end, and she wants no part of that. All along she had insisted that she would rather die than be helpless and dependent: "Someday I'm going to kill myself" (65); "I can't stand to live this way anymore. I'd rather die" (77); "I want to die" (198). By the last chapter she can no longer feed herself, dress herself, toilet herself, wash herself, speak, or use a computer. She manages to spell out on a letterboard this message to her husband: "I C-A-N-T T-A-L-K O-R W-A-L-K I D-O-N-T W-A-N-T T-O L-I-V-E L-I-K-E T-H-I-S A-N-Y M-O-RE" (197). In 2001, as Morton Kondracke's book about not saving Milly comes off the presses, things are desperate for Milly. She cannot swallow. If she does not get nourishment through a feeding tube, she will die. Morton asks Milly whether she wants the tube inserted. Despite her earlier resolutions that she would rather be dead than go that route, she now indicates that she wants to live. He has it inserted and she does live—if being bed-ridden and totally dependent can be called living. Three years later, on July 22, 2004, Milly dies.

Saving Milly does not paint a pretty picture of what may lie ahead for some people with Parkinson's. I recommend it for those who want to plan for the ugliness that may be around the bend.

B3. *When Parkinson's Strikes Early: Voices, Choices, Resources, and Treatment*, by Barbara Blake-Krebs, MA, and Linda Herman, MLS. Alameda, California: Hunter House, 2001. xiv + 270.

> "Above all, we hope our readers will come away with the understanding that there is life after Parkinson's. […] By working together as a community, we will beat this disease."

The primary authors of *When Parkinson's Strikes Early* are two women who were diagnosed in their mid-forties. Barbara Blake-Krebs, who worked at a radio station that she helped to found near Kansas City, was diagnosed in 1984 at age forty-four. A decade later Linda Herman, who worked as a librarian in Buffalo, was diagnosed at age forty-five. They searched for information about young-onset Parkinson's but found almost nothing. They tried attending support groups in their areas, but found in them few patients their own age. Late one night while she surfed the web, librarian Linda Herman stumbled upon the Parkinson's Information Exchange Network (PIEN) and there connected with Barbara Blake-Krebs and many others with young-onset Parkinson's. The two women decided to put together a book based on the e-mail stories that some seventy young-onset patients wrote on PIEN about their own experiences with the disease. They wove these stories together with what they knew of famous young-onset personages like Congressman Morris Udall, actor Michael J. Fox, and boxer Muhammed Ali. The purpose of their book, they said, was to offer

> patient-oriented information about physical symptoms at different stages of the disease and practical suggestions about coping with the changes and challenges PD brings into our lives. [...]
>
> Above all, we hope our readers will come away with the understanding that there is life after Parkinson's. It can be a devastating disease, indeed; however, by educating ourselves, taking an active role in treatment, seeking the support of others, and mostly by facing life with hope, we can meet the challenges. By working together as a community, we will beat this disease. (4–5)

Parkinson's, of course, ALWAYS strikes early—way too early. One is never ready for it. No one has ever said, "OK, Parkinson's, it's time. Come and strike me." But let's face it. It is one thing to have Parkinson's come around when we are in our sixties and seventies, when most of us are diagnosed. By then our marriages are mature, our children are grown, our careers are at or past their peaks, and we are probably at least thinking about making the transition into retirement. It is quite something else to have Parkinson's disease knock on our doors when we are in our twenties, thirties, and forties and calmly announce, "Hi. I'm here! I'm moving in. Get used to me, because you can't get rid of me and you can't run away from me! Now, then, where shall I put all this baggage I've brought along?"

The special problems that young-onset patients face are indeed daunting. Right from the start they have trouble getting an accurate diagnosis. Many doctors continue to think of Parkinson's as "an old people's disease" and tell their patients, "Well, it looks like Parkinson's, but you're too young to have that." Other problems have to do with truncated careers, financial planning, marital stresses, and parenting small children. As one young man from New Jersey wrote, "It really scares me when I think about how my life will be in a few years if we don't find a better treatment or cure for Parkinson's. I wonder if I will be able to teach my children how to ride a bike or dance at their weddings. I am scared about forced retirement before I'm financially stable" (35).

When Parkinson's Strikes Early is both an encouraging and a discouraging book. It is encouraging in that it shows that young-onset Parkinson people have found a way to use computer and web-based technology to find a sense of community with other people around the world who were diagnosed while young. Thanks to this technology, these patients no longer have to feel isolated by the fact that so few young-onset patients live near them. It is discouraging, however, in that in the sixteen years since this book was published in 2001, those same young-onset people have themselves grown older and are now experiencing essentially the "old people's disease" they once felt so distant from.

It is encouraging to see so much optimism in so many younger people with Parkinson's: "As we enter the twenty-first century, new treatment options are becoming available, and researchers now predict that a breakthrough is likely in five to ten years" (5). Later in the book a doctor with the disease writes that "the cure is not far off" (131). Later still, another patient writes that she sees good reason to "hope that in the relatively near future this beast of a disease will be tamed" (189). Another, referencing Muhammed Ali's boast that he floats like a butterfly but stings like a bee, writes that we are "ready to remove the sting from the bee of PD so that we can fly like butterflies" (201). It is discouraging, however, to realize that now, sixteen years later, the cure is still far off, that the breakthrough never broke through, that the beast is still beastly, that the PD bee still has its sting.

Though we never forget the circumstances in which we received the news that we have "an incurable degenerative disease," we are told early in the book, that "doctors can help their patients cope with the diagnosis by being truthful about the prognosis, encouraging patients to educate themselves, prescribing appropriate support services and therapies, and offering hope for the future" (21). It turns out, however, that there appears to be a contradiction between "being truthful about the prognosis" and "offering hope for the future."

I learned some interesting facts by readings this book. I learned, for example, that brain autopsies reveal that about a quarter of the people diagnosed with Parkinson's do not have it after all (20). I learned that Parkinson's is expensive: "The average annual cost of Parkinson's disease in the United States has been estimated at $25,000 per patient" (57). And I learned that, though Alzheimer's and Parkinson's are often grouped as similarly neurodegenerative, they are really opposites: "While Alzheimer's

destroys the mind, leaving the body functioning, Parkinson's destroys the
body's ability to function, imprisoning the mind inside" (8).

And I sometimes found myself nodding in silent agreement with
some of the statements Parkinson's patients emailed to the Parkinson's
Information Exchange Network. People who write about Parkinson's
often talk about the need to "fight" the disease. Two young-onset patients,
however, wrote of the futility of such fighting: "Mental attitude is half
the battle in dealing with PD. There is no use in fighting the disease, but
acceptance and determination keep many PD symptoms under control"
(41); "I had fought exhausting battles claiming occasional small victories in
an endless war I could not win instead of retreating, gradually, gracefully"
(47). Acceptance and grace—good words, those.

B4. *H.O.P.E: Four Keys to a Better Quality of Life for Parkinson's People,* by Hal Newsom. Seattle: Northwest Parkinson's Foundation, 2002. vii + 102 pp.

> "There are tens of thousands of Parkinson's
> People who are involved in vibrant lives. [...]
> They are not super heroes. They are ordinary
> people, with an un-ordinary health challenge."

One of the most engaging books about Parkinson's disease is that
written by Hal Newsom, a Seattle-based advertising executive.
Diagnosed at age 66, he lived with the disease for more than two decades.
He was active in the Northwest Parkinson's Foundation and helped start the
annual HOPE conference.

The success of Newsom's little book is due in part to its author's life-
experience in advertising. Like a good advertisement, it is short, focused,
well-written, personal, respectful, funny, not-too-technical, and packed
with stories that drive its points home. Hal Newsom ties what he says to
examples throughout. Instead of lecturing in the abstract about how to
react to the dreaded "You have Parkinson's" announcement from your
neurologist, he tells you about the reactions of Jack the disbeliever, Sue
the pro-activist, Carl the acceptor, and Bill the angry one. These examples
help us to see ourselves as most like Jack, Sue, Carl, or Bill, and help us to
understand that the most promising responses are those of Sue—"I've got it.

Now what am I going to do about it?" (10)—and Carl—"He didn't like the diagnosis but what could he do about it?" (11).

Much of the rest of the book is a direct answer to that question, what could Sue and Carl—that is, what can you—do about it? Hal Newsom refers not to "Parkinson's patients" but to "Parkinson's people." You need to think of yourself, he implies, not as a sick person with a debilitating disease but as a basically healthy person with a manageable disease:

> There are tens of thousands of Parkinson's People who are involved in vibrant lives—playing golf, skiing, swimming, walking, running, playing bridge, attending theater, operas, and symphonies, cooking, traveling, boating—even climbing mountains. These are people who are not fighting the disease but who are successfully living with it. They are not super heroes. They are ordinary people, with an unordinary health challenge. (8–9)

Many people advise fighting Parkinson's. They praise the people who fight the disease the hardest and longest. Hal Newsom is not one of those. He tells the story of Bill, "who fought the diagnosis of Parkinson's every step of the way." When he failed, Bill's only recourse was "to fight a little harder" (15). The way to get along best with this disease, Hal Newsom says, is to accept it, to recognize its power, to be glad it is not worse than it is, and to be grateful that help is readily available.

That word "help" brings us to the title of Hal Newsom's book, *H.O.P.E*—an acronym reminding people with Parkinson's of his four keys to a successful post-diagnosis life: Help, Optimism, Physician, and Exercise. These four keys serve to organize the book.

In the section on Help, Hal Newsom emphasizes that Parkinson's is not a disease that you should try to face alone. You owe it to your family—especially your spouse—to accept help in small ways at the start and in bigger ways as the disease moves along. Letting them help does not mean giving up your independence or burdening others, but it does mean consulting them from time to time, being open and honest about how you are feeling and managing, and letting them assist you in accordance with your needs and their abilities.

If you are still working, Help means letting your boss know about your diagnosis, being up front about how Parkinson's will affect your ability to do your job, and letting him or her know if you will need help.

Help means finding a congenial support group and attending meetings designed to give information and living proof that you are not alone. It is easy to convince yourself that only you have this disease and to feel increasingly isolated as the disease progresses. A support group and a couple of good friends who also have the disease will help you know that there are others who understand from the gut what you are experiencing.

The second letter in *H.O.P.E* stands for Optimism. It is easy enough to feel depressed if you have Parkinson's. You know that while medications can help alleviate some of the symptoms, none of those meds attack the disease itself, which churns on and on unchecked. How can you not feel depressed from time to time knowing that your disease will take away more and more of your independence with each passing year?

Hal Newsom offers some strategies that will help. He says that acceptance is crucial, admitting that "you can't control this disease" (48). If you accept up front "the idea that your body will not be the same as it was before," then you will be less likely to be depressed when your body changes as the disease progresses. Those who do not accept that and who "fight the disease every step of the way are formulating a pathway to frustration, depression, and unhappiness" (48).

Besides, Hal Newsome goes on, there are lots of reasons to feel positive about your disease. There are, for example, many medications that can help, and there is lots of information about the disease that helps you understand what is going on. You can also remind yourself of your many past triumphs and accomplishments. And you can set new goals for yourself, like biking to the next town or trekking to the top of a nearby mountain or hill. You can plan small and large adventures for yourself. You can refuse to quit. You can find ways to enjoy what you have now and not worry about what may— or may not—lie around the corner. You can laugh and make others laugh. You can stay active but also take time to rest when your body needs rest. You can refuse to hole up or to hide. You can volunteer to help others. But mostly you can accept what comes as it comes and not try to fight it: "if you elect to take on an optimistic attitude, you can find hundreds of ways to live with Parkinson's and enjoy a quality of life that is simply not possible with many other disorders" (64).

The third letter in *H.O.P.E* stands for Physician. Hal Newsom's point here is obvious enough: you need to find a movement disorder specialist you can trust, one who has a thorough knowledge of Parkinson's medications. These medications, applied at the right times and in the right doses, can do wonders for your quality of life. Again, acceptance is important: "Accept the idea that you'll probably be on medication for the remainder of your life. At first, that was a tough pill for me to swallow. But now it is such a part of me that I don't give it a second thought" (76).

The final letter in *H.O.P.E* stands for Exercise. Hal Newsom is particularly insistent on the need for people with Parkinson's to keep moving: " 'Use it or lose it' was never more true than with the Parkinson's crowd" (87). He particularly advocates aggressive activities like running and biking, but realizes that they are not for everyone. He suggests that you find activities that you enjoy—walking, swimming, tennis, golf, whatever: "The point is, no matter how non-athletic you have been in the past, you absolutely must undertake an exercise program if you have Parkinson's" (92). And as always with Hal Newsom, the key word is acceptance: "Parkinson's is such a part of me that the inconveniences of the disease seem natural. As though I were selected for some strange reason to awaken each day for the rest of my life with the reality that my body has dramatically changed. I can't correct that. But I can accept it" (102).

Hal Newsom's book is a plain-spoken and calming introduction to a frightening new reality for people newly diagnosed with Parkinson's and for their families. Hal Newsom himself died in 2015, but his *H.O.P.E* lives on.

B4. *Lucky Man: A Memoir*, by Michael J. Fox. New York: Hyperion, 2002. 260 pp.

> "PD's brutal assumption of authority over more and more aspects of life makes you appreciate all those areas where you still have sovereignty."

Michael J. Fox was at the top of his acting career. For his portrayal of Alex Keaton in the television sitcom *Family Ties* he had won three consecutive Emmys (1986, 1987, 1988) and a Golden Globe (1989). He was already famous for his portrayal of Marty McFly in *Back to the Future*, the highest-grossing movie of 1985. The millions were rolling in. He had recently (1988) married and he and his lovely wife had had their first child.

And then one morning in November of 1990, while he was in Gainesville, Florida, making a film called *Doc Hollywood*, he noticed, as he came out of his customary hangover, that his left little finger had a mind of its own: "It was trembling, twitching, auto-animated" (2). Had he slept on that hand in some weird way? Was it a signal that he was drinking too much, an early-warning delirium tremens of some sort? He made a series of fists with his hands and shook them out. The tremor was still there.

We all go through a period of denial when we first see signs that we may have Parkinson's. It is partly that we don't know much about this disease, partly that we don't want to know anything about it. We think we cannot have it: we never handled Agent Orange; we have no Parkinson's in our family; we are morally upright, for the most part, and have done nothing to deserve this kind of punishment; we are far too young to have this disease; and so on.

With Parkinson's, however, denial is at best a temporary escape. Whatever was causing the thirty-year-old Michael J. Fox's left pinkie to wander around was soon causing other fingers on his left hand also to go their separate ways. His denial lasted about a year. Michael finally agreed to try a low dose of L-dopa. If it helped, then he would know that he had Parkinson's. It helped. Thirty minutes after he took half a pill, his tremor disappeared for almost five hours. "The bad news was obvious: here was yet another confirmation I had Parkinson's disease. The good news was now I could hide it" (150). And hide it he did. Telling only a few members of his family and a few trusted friends that he had Parkinson's, he delayed going public with the information until seven years later.

Michael J. Fox tried to find out why he had the disease. Was he, he wondered, being punished for his storybook rise to wealth and fame as an actor? Was Parkinson's "the cosmic price I had to pay for my success" (118–19)? He never found the answer to his "Why me?" Few of us do.

Although the two Parkinson's events—finding out about his disease and letting others find out about it—structure Michael J. Fox's memoir, *Lucky Man* is not predominantly about Parkinson's. Most of the first half is about Michael J. Fox's growing up in Canada, his family, his decision to drop out of high school and move to Hollywood to take a shot at a professional acting career, his uncertain start in acting, his years of poverty and debt, his hard work, and his lucky breaks.

Meanwhile, he tried another kind of medication, alcohol. He describes the time his three-year-old son Sam woke him up out of a mid-day hangover. That event, and his disgusted wife's question, "Is this what you want?" made him realize that it was not at all what he wanted:

> You hear stories of utter financial ruin, horrendous car wrecks, injury, and death, prison sentences, wrecked marriages, degradation, and humiliation far beyond anything I'd ever experienced. But as long as I continued to drink, any one of those fates could have been mine. (160)

He finally gave up drinking:

I couldn't do anything about P.D., but alcohol was different: here at least I had a choice, and that day I made it. Helping me to make that choice was the first thing I'd actually be grateful to Parkinson's for. Part of the disease's "gift" is a certain stark clarity about the rest of your life. P.D.'s brutal assumption of authority over more and more aspects of life makes you appreciate all those areas where you still have sovereignty. (160)

Early in his book Michael J. Fox provocatively announces that "these last ten years of coming to terms with my disease [have been] the best ten years of my life—not in spite of my illness, but because of it." He speaks of the disease as a "gift." He readily admits that while some gifts just keep on giving, this one "just keeps on taking." And while he is fully aware that no one would ever choose to receive this gift of "relentless assault and accumulating damage," he insists that being forced to deal with it has "profoundly enriched" his life: "That's why I consider myself a lucky man" (5). He liked the person Parkinson's disease made him: "If you were to rush into this room right now announce that you had struck a deal [...] in which the ten years since my diagnosis could be magically taken away, traded for ten more years as the person I was before—I would, without a moment's hesitation, tell you to take a hike" (6).

There is much to admire in Michael J. Fox. He had the gumption to rise from poverty to the pinnacle of his profession. He found the good in a bad diagnosis. He refused to let a miserable disease make him miserable. He escaped the escape into alcoholism. He admitted his shortcomings and laughed—and makes us laugh—at his stumbles.

Lucky us. We are lucky that Michael J. Fox's fame gave Parkinson's a more public face than it had before. We are lucky that he has used some of his millions to establish a foundation that continues to support research that we all hope will lead to a cure for Parkinson's. But we are lucky mostly because he has shown us one man's way to find the good in what at first looks only bad.

B6. *The First Year—Parkinson's Disease: An Essential Guide for the Newly Diagnosed,* **by Jackie Hunt Christensen. New York: Marlowe, 2005. xxi + 335 pp.**

> "When we Parkies forget where we put our car keys, or our reason for going from one room to another, we often panic and assume we are developing dementia."

Jackie Hunt Christensen was diagnosed with Parkinson's in 1998 at the age of thirty-four, not long after her second child was born. She is pretty sure that she contracted the disease years earlier, because she grew up in a rural area where the soybean farmers routinely used strong fertilizers to stimulate the growth of the soybeans and strong herbicides to control the weeds in their fields. She spent several summers as a teenager working in those fields and even spraying them with the herbicides. Then, in 1988 she worked as an environmental river tour guide on the Mississippi. In one of these tours she found herself wading, without protective rubber boots, in the effluent from a sewage disposal plant in St. Louis.

Her book is a part of a series of *First Year* books published by Marlowe. There is one on *The First Year—Type 2 Diabetes,* one on *The First Year— Multiple Sclerosis,* one on *The First Year—Fibromyalgia,* and so on. In *The First year—Parkinson's Disease,* Jackie Christensen leads us through the seven days of the first week after our diagnosis.

On Day 1 she tells us what Parkinson's disease is and how it is diagnosed. On Day 2 she tells us about the early symptoms of the disease and how it affects the brain. On Day 3 she describes the most common medicines used to treat Parkinson's and about what to expect when we take carbidopa/levodopa, the most commonly prescribed medicine for Parkinson's. On Day 4 she talks about hereditary and environmental causes of Parkinson's. On Day 5 her subject is the physical and mental effects of Parkinson's, on Day 6 it is depression and coming to terms with the diagnosis, and on Day 7 it is telling others about our diagnosis and drug therapies for anxiety and depression. That gets us to the "first-week milestone" and ends the day-by-day chapters.

Then Jackie Christensen moves us to topics of Weeks 2, 3, and 4: complementary therapies, the "gifts" that come with having Parkinson's, and the need to take care of our care partners. With that fourth week we reach the "first-month milestone." After that she takes us through chapters devoted not to a day or a week, but a whole month at a time. After eleven of these one-month chapters, we reach the "first-year milestone" and the book is finished, except for appendices, notes, a glossary, a list of resources, and a bibliography.

The First Year—Parkinson's Disease packs in a lot of useful information, though I find the day-week-month chapter divisions to be somewhat artificial. I also find it sometimes misleading that she feels the need to divide each of the twenty-one chapters (seven days, three weeks, and eleven months) into two parts, the first on "Living" the second on "Learning." In the chapter on Month 7, for example, the "Living" part is about exercise while the "Learning" part is about traveling. For Month 8 the "Living" part is about sexuality while the "Learning" part is about sleep. It all begins to sound like an arbitrary outline in which all that we need to know about Parkinson's in the first year can be shoe-horned into forty-two sections, twenty-one on "Living" and twenty-one on "Learning." Are living and learning really all that different?

And do we really need to know in the first year of our diagnosis about the risk of dementia?:

> Forgetfulness is one of the first signs of dementia, so when we Parkies forget where we put our car keys, or our reason for going from one room to another, we often panic and assume we are developing dementia. [...] The good news is not everyone who has PD will develop dementia. [...] The likelihood of dementia increases with age (12.4 percent in people of age fifty to fifth-nine, rising to 68.7 percent in patients over eighty). (223)

That may be true, but why do we need to know it in the ninth month after diagnosis?

Indeed, I question the fundamental premise of the book: that the emphasis should be on the first year after diagnosis. The first year is the easiest for people with Parkinson's. In the first year the symptoms are slight and usually not obvious to others. Many of us do not even take medicine for the first year. What we really need is help knowing how to manage the last year. By then the meds are losing their ability to help us, the side effects are in full evidence, our off-times are longer, and it is clear that no cure that could help us is in the pipeline.

Mentioning a cure brings me to Jackie Christensen's cheerfully inclusive introduction:

> I want to begin by expressing my admiration for you, as a newly
> diagnosed or recently diagnosed person with Parkinson's disease, for
> having the courage to learn more about this intrusion into your life.
> Parkinson's disease will affect how you live your life from now until
> a cure is found or you pass away. (xv)

She mentions a cure for Parkinson's again a couple of pages later: "We are
living in an age where new research is being done every day to find the
cause(s) and cure for PD and to develop treatments to help us cope until
a cure is available" (xx). The closing salutation in her introduction again
mentions a cure: "Yours in the struggle to find the cause and cure" (xxi). At
the other end of the book, the title of the second or "Learning" segment of
Month 11 is entitled "Help to Find a Cure." I am not sure it is wise to speak
as if a cure is imminent or inevitable. Is it wise to encourage the newly-
diagnosed "Parkies" (why do I gag on that term?) to wait for a cure that has
been eluding us for two centuries, ever since Dr. Parkinson first described
the "shaking palsy"? Would it not be wiser to help people learn to live
productively and peacefully with the fact that there is no known cure for
their disease?

B7. *Stop Parkin' and Start Livin': Reversing the Symptoms of Parkinson's Disease*, by John C. Coleman, ND. South Yarra, Australia: Michelle Anderson Publishing, 2005. vi + 341 pp.

> "Recovery takes a long time—at least four years
> and maybe much more."

In 1995 John Coleman was diagnosed with late-stage Parkinson's disease.
Having already begun studying for a degree in naturopathy, he decided
not to take the Western-style medicines that neurologists prescribed for
his condition. He decided instead to try a number of less "conservative"
options. Three years later, having completed his Diploma of Naturopathy
from the Australian College of Natural Medicine in Melbourne, he declared
himself symptom-free and began seeing clients of his own. What he offered
them—besides the sympathy of a co-sufferer with Parkinson's disease—was

the possibility of getting better. He puts it this way early in *Stop Parkin'
and Start Livin'*: "I offered hope of recovery—not because I offered to cure
them (I can't), but because I had recovered and understood pretty well how
I had reached my state of health" (8).

That statement introduces a key distinction between two words that
many people consider to be nearly synonymous: recovery and cure. For
many people, to say "I recovered from prostate cancer" means pretty
much the same thing as "I was cured of prostate cancer." When pressed,
these people might say that one can "recover" without the intervention of
a physician, as in "by the weekend I had fully recovered from my cold,"
whereas to be "cured" suggests both the agency of a doctor and a more
permanent fix. To recover from a cold is temporary; the chances are good
that you will get another cold within a year. To be "cured" suggests that a
physician intervened medically or surgically to stop the illness, and that it
will not return.

John Coleman draws a fundamental distinction between a cure for
Parkinson's and recovery from it. There is no cure for Parkinson's, he says,
by which he means that there is no pill, treatment, or surgery that will stop
the disease and make patients all better again. There is, however, a way
to recover from Parkinson's, by which he means to improve and even get
free of the symptoms of the disease. But he seems at times uncertain of his
meanings. If there is indeed no cure for Parkinson's, what are we to make of
his statement that "there are no incurable diseases, just incurable people"?
(13).

He gives six "rules for recovery":

    1. There is no easy way to recover. There is no magic pill or
miracle therapy that will suddenly remove all symptoms.

    2. The level of symptom reversal achieved depends on disease
severity, age, concomitant ailments, damage from drugs, chemicals,
injury or surgery, and the level of dedication the client and their
carer(s) bring to the recovery process.

    3. Recovery takes a long time—at least four years and maybe
much more.

    4. The recovery process is multi-faceted and involves a number
of therapies plus, most importantly, individual effort.

    5. Full recovery can only occur if each person is treated as they

deserve—i.e. as a wonderful, beautiful, complex creation by the Supreme Spirit (God, the Universe, etc.) who made all things. [...]

6. Recovery requires dedicated, frustrating work on the part of the client, the carer(s), and the practitioners. (9–10)

It is not hard to understand why John Coleman has had some difficulty gaining widespread approval or support for his approach. Let's assume that a woman named Madeline has been diagnosed with Parkinson's disease. After she reads John Coleman's book, her thinking process might go something like this:

> Gosh, it sounds hard. He keeps saying that there is no easy way to recover and that I have to be ready to do dedicated, frustrating work for a long time. Do I really want to risk so much for such uncertain reward? Who is accountable if, after years of effort, I am not getting any better? The way he puts it, I will have been entirely at fault because I have not worked hard or long enough, or have not been "dedicated" enough. Besides, I am not sure what is implied by the statement that "recovery can only occur if each person is treated as they deserve"? How do I know if I am treated as I deserve? And what are the implications of that Supreme Spirit he speaks of? I also wonder about John Coleman's past success rate. He says in his book that his methods have proven successful in "my own experience and that of a very few individuals around the world" (8). A couple of pages later he admits that his methods have led to "only one claim of complete recovery (me)" (10). He says that "many people" in his program "are now being rewarded with improving health," but that sounds pretty vague. He says that "some will fully recover from their symptoms of Parkinson's disease as I did" (11). But what about the others, the ones who do not recover? Besides, I am kind of concerned that there is some question about whether John Coleman's initial diagnosis was accurate. If he never had true Parkinson's disease to start with, does it make any sense for him to claim to have recovered from it?

The various Madelines in the world will need to decide for themselves whether to go with traditional Western medicine, with an alternative approach like John Coleman's, or with some combination of the two. Those who want to cast their lot with Western medicine will find much to interest them and help them in *Stop Parkin' and Start Livin'*. John Coleman has much to say about what foods to eat and what foods to avoid, about the importance of water and exercise, about the importance of relaxation and meditation, about the importance of social contacts. Would it not be possible for Madeline to learn from both approaches? John Coleman seems to want to preclude that possibility by demonizing Western neurologists.

It does not help his cause for John Coleman to be so openly suspicious of Western-style neurologists. What is gained by his telling his readers that, while there are "many wonderful, caring doctors in the world,"

> some specializing in treatment of the aged or neuro-degenerative disorders feel that they can ride roughshod over the needs and wishes of their clients. As many people suffering from these disorders are old, debilitated, inhibited in mobility and, often, have difficulty with communication, it is easy for practitioners to assert control and impose their ideas on clients. (7)

What is gained by characterizing the patients of Western-style neurologists as the victims of bloodless doctor-machines?:

> In the rigmarole of appointments, referrals, tests, scans, examinations and form filling, the patients lose their right to exist as an individual, and become a "case" for each practitioner, to be defined by data, treated by statistical outcome, and lost in the cauldron of mechanistic medicine. (46)

Few patients will feel that their neurologists are such people as that or that they themselves are lost in such a cauldron. It will be hard for Madeline, in the face of such negativity, to feel positive about her chances for recovery if she signs on for this alternative approach to her Parkinson's.

B8. *Shake Well before Use: A Walk around Britain's Coastline,* by Tom Isaacs. King's Lynn, Norfolk: Cure for Parkinson's Press, 2007. 335 pp.

> "Parkinson's was the stuff of nightmares, except that when I woke up from this strange and distant reverie, the reality of my situation would be even worse."

Tom Isaacs will be familiar to anyone who attended the Northwest Parkinson's Foundation's 2015 HOPE conference in Seattle. He was the keynote speaker whose intrusive dyskinesia as he spoke did not prevent his audience from hearing his inspiring message, from laughing at his corny jokes, and from applauding his closing song-and-dance.

Shake Well before Use is Tom Isaacs's detailed account of his year-long walk around the coastline of Britain. The book is many things: a photo-illustrated travelogue, a tribute to a deceased father and a loving mother, a fund-raising manual, a love story, a saga of a young man struggling to learn how to accept the questionable gifts that Parkinson's delivered to him. In this review I focus especially on the last of those.

Tom Isaacs was diagnosed with Parkinson's at the unripe young age of twenty-seven. His reaction to the news will sound familiar to many of us:

> Parkinson's was the stuff of nightmares, except that when I woke up from this strange and distant reverie, the reality of my situation would be even worse. [...] Yesterday I had potential. [...] Yesterday I had the best of my life ahead of me. [...] I wanted it to be yesterday again. (xix–xx)

He knew, however, that yesterday was gone forever, and all he had to work with was tomorrow—and of course today.

At first he tried to hide his Parkinson's, but as the shaking got worse, that approach proved to be both isolating and futile: "But what could I do? I felt helpless. I wanted to take Parkinson's on; compete with it; fight it; anything other than just wait for it to gradually take hold" (16). He decided that, rather than hide his shaking, he would "go public and reveal my illness to everyone. I would fight it now. The question was how" (13). His answer to that "how" was a decision to raise money to support scientific research leading to a cure for Parkinson's by "Coastin' "—that is, by walking around the perimeter of Britain in the most public way possible: "Instead of hiding the fact that I had Parkinson's disease, I forced myself to allow people to see me shaking so that both they and I would be comfortable with it" (70). He enlisted the help of friends and professional public relations people, and on April 11, 2002, at age thirty-three, he started his twelve-month hike by walking east from London with the aid of a walking stick that he named Ewan.

Tom Isaacs took the title of his book from a little song that he wrote to be sung to the tune of Billy Joel's "You're Always a Woman to Me." Here is the opening stanza:

> *To the fridge in the morning, I reach for my juice*
> *There's a sign on the top says "Shake well before use*
> *But I don't need instructions, I have expertise*
> *Completely superfluous message with Parkies disease.* (117)

Tom Isaacs's sense of humor helped him to deal with the many hardships—some of them dangerous—on the 4500-mile journey in which he climbed the three tallest mountains in Britain and wore out five pairs of hiking boots. Sometimes he got lost on poorly-marked footpaths. Sometimes the weather was foggy, rainy, or bitterly cold. Sometimes he was eaten alive by armies of bloodthirsty mosquitoes (he calls them midges). Sometimes he had to make his way through barbed wire or along crumbling cliff-trails. Sometimes the pain in his legs was so great that he could scarcely stand it. Sometimes his meds did not work the way they were supposed to. For example, when he had waded halfway across the River Borgie at the upper end of Torrisdale Bay, his dopamine suddenly quit working and he froze up:

> It can be that quick. One moment I am a fully functional human being, the next, almost totally incapacitated. [...] My balance was suddenly non-existent. I clung on to Ewan, my stick, for support as if it was my only lifeline and I made my way, inch by inch, across the slippery rocks at the bottom of the stream. My journey to the center of the stream had been about three seconds. The second half of the trip probably took sixty times as long. (135–36)

The reactions of those whom Tom Isaacs encountered on his journey were usually sympathetic, but not always sensitive. The proprietress of a bed-and-breakfast refused during one of his more kinetic shaking bouts to give him extra time to pack his gear and check out. And then there was the bloke he encountered at a pub in Hart. When the man found out that Tom Isaacs had Parkinson's, he said, "Oh, I'm really sorry, mate. You must feel awful. I mean, basically, you're completely f***ked" (86).

About halfway through his journey Tom Isaacs made the startling discovery that he had never felt better:

> I felt fulfilled. It dawned on me that fulfillment has nothing to do with success, wealth, or reward, nor health for that matter. Fulfillment was about making the most of my capabilities and concentrating on the things that seemed important to me. Coastin' was giving me an outdoor life, a goal, a course, and a life-enriching experience. It was all I wanted. [...] I had truly found the answer to my Parkinson's. Perhaps out of its remorseless campaign to ruin my life, I had seen a way to find out not just acceptance, but even fulfillment. Perhaps, instead of fighting Parkinson's, I could use its energy and redirect it to really positive effect. Perhaps the rest of my life could be lived not despite Parkinson's, but because of it. (146)

Tom Isaacs's walk generated some £350,000 in donations and sponsorships. That money was given to researchers seeking to find a cure for Parkinson's. That money, that research, may someday lead to a cure. But Tom Isaacs's lessons about finding fulfillment through Parkinson's, rather than merely in spite of it, can perhaps help us all right now.

B9. *Surviving Adversity: Living with Parkinson's Disease*, by Gord Carley, 2007. iv + 171 pp.

> "Try not to waste a day or an hour or even a moment of your life. Celebrate. Have fun. Enjoy the journey."

G ord Carley says little about how he gathered the twenty-eight first-person "profiles" that he presents in *Surviving Adversity*, but to judge from what he published in his book, I am supposing that his letter of invitation went something like this:

Dear _____:

I have learned that you are one of the 1.5 million people in North America who have been diagnosed with Parkinson's. I want to publish a series of first-person profiles written by a select few of those. I would very much like it if you would write your story for publication.

I have in mind an autobiographical essay of around 2500 words, more or less, in which you share your story: who you are, how and at what age you first found out you have Parkinson's, how you reacted to news of the diagnosis, what you have learned about the disease and yourself as a result of your experience with the disease, and what advice you would offer to others who have recently been diagnosed.

Our target audience is newly-diagnosed Parkinson's patients who know almost nothing about the disease and who are variously worried, puzzled, shocked, or depressed by the news. I am hoping that, taken together, the various profiles I publish will give them useful strategies for coping with the disease....

Gord Carley tells us nothing about how many such letters he wrote, how many individuals sent him their profiles, or how many he accepted. All we know is that among them were many Canadians and at least some famous personages like Olympic cyclist Davis Phinney and U.S. Attorney General Janet Reno. The stories are as varied as the men and women who wrote them, and so is the advice. In this short review I cut to the chase by quoting a few of the pithy bits of advice the writers offer. Most of that advice tended to involve six topics: knowing that we have the power to choose, staying active, finding the good, having a sunny outlook, remembering to laugh, and thinking about a cure.

Knowing that we have the power to choose

Pat Hull: "Worry is a waste of time and energy. You just have to look to the future and deal with it. When something happens to you that isn't pleasant, you can choose to continue on, stand up and do things and have a good time, or you can quit and wilt. It is definitely your choice." (13–14)

Patty Meehan: "I made a conscious choice that I am going to live a full life with Parkinson's and that I will not let it become an excuse." (100)

Staying active

Tom O'Donnell: "It is easier to handle Parkinson's by doing things and keeping active than by sitting in a chair and being depressed. Never ever give up. Parkinson's may steal your mind and your body—but will never touch your heart and your soul. Quitting is the harder way out." (113)

Cheerie Zaun: "You can't sit in a recliner and feel sorry for yourself. You have to get out of the chair and live life. Do something about it. You have to keep trying." (119)

Finding the good

Janet Sinke: "In a way, getting Parkinson's has been one of my greatest blessings because it has given me an opportunity to look at life from a different mountain and to go down paths I would not have been on otherwise. Try not to waste a day or an hour or even a moment of your life. Celebrate. Have fun. Enjoy the journey." (31)

John Ball: "Parkinson's is not a tragedy. Events happen in life. [...] The solution to problems comes from within yourself, not from outside." (24)

Having a sunny outlook

Knolton Nash: "It's important to have a sunny outlook. [...] With Parkinson's, you just have to cope with it and get on with it." (18–19)

Robbie Tucker: "I have to have a positive outlook on life because there is no reason why I shouldn't." (155)

Raul Yzaguirre: "Having a positive attitude is the most important thing. Parkinson's provides a new way to learn and grow." (36)

Janet Reno: "If you fail at something, pick yourself up and try again. A sense of hope, held in a realistic way, is something that all Parkinson's patients can develop and share." (161)

Remembering to laugh

Bill Commans: "If you can laugh at yourself and your clumsiness and not curse every time you stumble, it makes things easier. [...] When I can't move, I just try to laugh and remind myself that I have Parkinson's and I can't do too much to get rid of it, so I might as well accept it." (47–48)

Chris Olsen: "I believe the positive things are there—you just have to look for them. I try to keep laughter close to the surface—I think we all need to find the humor that is around us." (53)

Irv Popkin: "It is important to not self-obsess. You need to smile and snap out of it. I like to make people laugh." (59)

Magda Schiff: "You need to see the humor in life." (142)

Thinking about a cure

Steve Bohannon: "I feel strongly that there is a cure on the horizon, and for a lot of diseases that cannot be said. I consider myself lucky because I am young enough that I feel I will have many Parkinson's-free years ahead of me when the cure is discovered." (71)

John Thomas: "It is important to be realistic that a cure for Parkinson's may be more than five years away. I have seen a lot of 'five years' go by already. [...] That being said, I think it is important to look on the bright side—maybe they will find something in the near future." (83)

David Heydrick: "We receive reports from the media that a cure is near, yet it seems that we are constantly being disappointed. Ultimately, we keep going—and I am sure that eventually our persistence will be rewarded and we will raise our arms in victory!" (96)

Davis Phinney: "My advice is to become as knowledgeable as you can about Parkinson's but not to become obsessed about when a cure or medical wonder is going to happen. The medical wonder that you can affect is in your daily approach to managing your disease and that includes both physical and mental aspects. Focus on the positive, acknowledge your victories, and make every day a good day." (5)

We might have hoped for a summary or synthesizing discussion of the various views presented by the twenty-eight contributors. But Gord Carley provides none. We might have hoped for a more ambitious title than *Surviving Adversity*, since some of the contributors seem to think it is possible to do more than merely "survive" Parkinson's.

B10. *I Have Parkinson's But Parkinson's Does Not Have Me!*, by Leif Ögård, translated from the Swedish by David Mel Paul. Höllviken, Sweden: Copyright by Leif Ögård, 2008. 165 pp.

> "From the very moment I decided to fight Parkinson's disease I have stubbornly insisted that I am healthy—not sick."

A Swedish business man named Leif Ögård, born in 1942, was at the top of his game when, in 1987, at age forty-five, he was told by a neurologist that he had Parkinson's disease and that he would so rapidly lose his ability to move that in five years he would be confined to a wheelchair. He was devastated. He allowed himself to sink deeper and deeper into despair. He gradually worked his way out of his hopelessness and began to think more positively about his life and his disease. Fourteen years later he had proved that first neurologist wrong by still functioning successfully. His business was a success, he was a loving member of his family, and he was emphatically not confined to a wheelchair. He had found a way, by using levodopa carefully and by keeping a positive attitude, to keep Parkinson's at bay. He told others about the reasons for his amazing success, but no one was much impressed. He wanted to help others by writing a book about his experience, but no one gave him any encouragement. "Hold Parkinson's disease at bay with positive thinking?" "Nonsense," they seemed to say.

In 2001 Leif Ögård read Donald B. Caine's article in Science magazine, "Expectations and Dopamine Release—Mechanisms of the Placebo Effect in Parkinson's Disease." In that article, Caine

> presented evidence that patients themselves could affect (increase) their own production of the signal substance dopamine, the indisputable substance whose deficiency in the body creates Parkinson's disease. Fantastic! Now at last it had been proven that a person's attitude and mind-set and a person's own will could affect the progress of the disease and thereby its influence on our lives! (12)

Encouraged by Caine's findings, Leif Ögård decided to write his book.

His audience is people who have been diagnosed with Parkinson's and are deeply discouraged about their prognosis:

> My intention is to make this a hopeful book. For even though I describe a highly demanding way to achieve an active and good life full of eager enjoyment, I guarantee that the result will be worth every scintilla of effort—several times over! And you need not worry whether you can do it, because you can. If I can, so can you! This is a book for you who are trying to see the possibilities in place of the problems. It is written both for you who already are optimistic and also for you who are trying to find the grounds to become so. Both of you will be richly rewarded. (13)

The main substance of Leif Ögård's book can be summarized in eight statements:

1. Accept responsibility. There are two pathways out of the valley of Parkinson's, one he calls "Help-Me Street" and the other he calls "Help-Myself Way." The second is the one you should take, even though it is the "more winding and difficult one" (21).

2. Believe in your own power. If you believe that your thoughts can influence your health, they can; if you don't, they won't: "Believe you are going to feel better, and you shall. […] Believe you are going to feel worse, and you shall" (42).

3. Think positively. A positive outlook about your health pays off: "If you think only negatively, your life is going to become negative" (45). "From the very moment I decided to fight Parkinson's disease I have stubbornly insisted that I am healthy—not sick" (96).

4. Believe in the future. Take your levodopa as prescribed, but never give up hope. Just as a cure for tuberculosis was discovered in the 1950s, so a cure for Parkinson's may soon be found: "Considering the present headlong pace of development I cannot help but believe that the solution to the nearly two-centuries-old puzzle of Parkinson's is right around the corner" (64).

5. Your mind has great power, even over the health of your body. "Eight years ago I decided that I had really had enough of colds. They disturbed too much my body's utilization of the dopamine medicine. No sooner said than done. I visualized in a picture that my immune system took care of all cold virus attacks! […] I have not had a cold one single time during the last five years!" (68)

6. See your Parkinson's disease as an opportunity. Instead of whining about your disease, learn from it, grow from it: "The struggle in itself, against Parkinson and for life, gives you an unbelievable chance for personal development" (81).

7. Make Mr. Parkinson your friend. He will soon be vanquished by a cure. When that happens, you may even find that you miss him: "Mr. Parkinson, once my uninvited guest, had become a traveling companion! [...] These last years I have found more and more ways to joke with Mr. Parkinson, and he has returned the favor. [...] I think he is simply beginning to realize that his time is approaching its end" (144).

8. Laugh. Find something to laugh at, someone to laugh with: "Seek out happy people! Make others laugh" (145).

Leif Ögård ends his book with a self-satisfied sigh. He set out "to write the book I myself so desperately needed twenty years ago. I have written it for you. [...] I know my book is going to help people gain a better life" (147). I hope his book does cheer people up and help them find a better life. It will no doubt do so for readers who share his super-positive approach to Parkinson's disease, readers who share his optimism that the disease will soon be conquered, his belief that a cure for Parkinson's is just around the corner, his faith that the worst is past and the best is yet to come.

B11. *Parkinson's Disease: Looking Down the Barrel*, by Richard Secklin. Milwaukee, Wisconsin: Nettfit Publishing, 2010. 78 pp.

> "But now I am losing everything. I have Parkinson's disease and my symptoms are steadily advancing."

When Richard Secklin, a career law enforcement officer in Texas, was diagnosed with Parkinson's disease in 2003, his life took a nosedive. His wife divorced him. He began using marijuana. He quit his job. He almost committed suicide. His teenage son suggested that he move back to Milwaukee where his daughters from a previous marriage lived. He did. In Milwaukee he tried several jobs, lost them, and fell deeply into debt. Then his life began to turn around. He applied for Social Security disability benefits and got them. He found his way to a VA hospital, where he was treated for depression, bipolar disease, and Parkinson's. He fell in love and married again. He began to enjoy his various children and grandchildren. Life was much better.

The subtitle refers to the author's contemplating suicide:

> I am hysterically crying as I look down the barrel of my Glock 17. I am thinking, my temple or in my mouth? [...]
>
> I am sitting at the edge of my bed sweating. My hand is shaking; my finger twitching on the trigger. My life flashes before me.
>
> I had survived psychological and physical events before. I had endured infidelity and divorce. I had survived a broken neck and had my chest opened up for the removal of a large cyst.
>
> But now I am losing everything. I have Parkinson's disease and my symptoms are steadily advancing. (8–9)

Parkinson's Disease: Looking Down the Barrel is a short book of only seventy-eight double-spaced pages. It reads—very quickly—like a cross between a suicide note and a letter thanking God for his many blessings. We all have a story to tell about our feelings and dealings with Parkinson's, our down times and our lift times. It apparently helped Richard Secklin to write his story down. I am not sure it will help others to read that story.

B12. *The Unexpected Journey: Living on the Edge of Life's Promise,* by George L. Johnston. Greenville, South Carolina: Ambassador International, 2010. 135 pp.

> "For those who struggle with PD, all I can say about my journey to this point is that there is still abundant joy, grace, and consolation to be found."

George Johnson, a California lawyer at the top of his game, was diagnosed with Parkinson's disease in 1994 when he was forty-three years old. Following the diagnosis he engaged for many years in compulsive gambling that cost him his job, ended his marriage, alienated his children, and left him financially destitute. During that difficult time he took daily walks during which he composed short aphorisms that he called "lodestones." He was eventually invited by the Parkinson's Association of Northern California to write a monthly column for their newsletter. Entitled "Views from the Park Bench," the column was supposed to be an insider's guide to the disease. George Johnston eventually published his "Park Bench" contributions, along with the aphorisms he calls lodestone aphorisms, as a slender book called *The Unexpected Journey*. It is a wise, thoughtful, honest, modest, and eloquent little book that deserves to be read carefully and often.

In *The Unexpected Journey*, Johnston offers useful information and advice to others with Parkinson's. He tells us, for example, why he hates the diminutive term "Parkie" and resents being asked to generalize about what people with Parkinson's believe:

> I was sitting in a group discussing health care reform (haven't we all?) when someone looked at me and said, "And what does the Parkie contingent have to add to this debate?" [...] If you are going to ask my opinion as part of a group, ask about the group that brought strength and adult responsibilities to my life, not the group that sends signals to everyone that I may be weak or incapable of playing a full-contact sport. (33, 35)

He sings the praises of deep-brain stimulation: "Each day I mourn for those who for whatever reason are not able to have this procedure done or who have had the procedure done but have not obtained the same measure of benefits that I have" (76–77). But even after DBS, life is still a struggle:

> Living with Parkinson's for me is a daily struggle of ego with reality. My ego says I am still that young, vibrant, I-can-meet-any-challenge man that I was when I was thirty. Reality says that I am a fifty-eight-year-old man with Parkinson's disease, who has had brain surgery to have metal rods implanted in my brain to alleviate most of the motor problems that I had to deal with pre-surgery, who still needs to take medication in order to have my body move at all. (59)

As a result of his experience helping victims of the Katrina hurricane catastrophe in New Orleans, he offers eminently sensible advice about preparing for a similar disaster in our own neighborhoods. We should make sure, he says, that we have at hand in a watertight container a full change of clothes, a full month's supply of our medications, information about what diseases or conditions the medications are for, the names and contact information of the doctors who prescribed them, and instructions about dosages and schedules for administering them: "Just think for a moment what it would be like if you were alone in a disastrous situation, scared, running out of medication, without a change of clothes, and with no ability to communicate immediately to first responders pertinent medical information about your condition. It is not a pretty sight" (85–86).

He suggests that people with Parkinson's are so susceptible to dangerously compulsive behaviors like shopping and gambling because of the payoff in dopamine:

> You don't shop compulsively because you want the objects, you shop because you crave the additional dopamine that the activity causes your brain to produce. You don't become a compulsive gambler because you want the money, you do it because you want the sweet feeling of relief that passes through your body when you get the "hit" of additional dopamine. (101)

He suggests that people with Parkinson's consider getting a service dog. His own dog, Akua, provides him with constant companionship, helps pull him up steep hills, helps him find his way through crowded spaces, and helps him get unstuck when he freezes or spends too much time on the couch.

George Johnson advises full disclosure: "after being diagnosed with PD you hide the destructive aspects of your behavior from your doctor, spouse, or friends at your extreme peril" (103).

Like everyone who has Parkinson's, Johnston wondered why and how he got it: genetics? head-battering? pesticides? the FDA? the military? At first he wanted to know who to blame, who to punish, but he outgrows that petty pursuit: "You can blame and stay stuck in the past, or you can forgive and resolve and move forward to the future" (113). He offers wise advice to people with Parkinson's, to people who care for us, and to the rest of the world:

> For those who struggle with PD, all I can say about my journey to this point is that there is still abundant joy, grace, and consolation to be found: the mine is just deeper and hauling the gold into the light of day takes a bit longer.
>
> For those who care for someone with PD, try to be a patient, positive companion. I know that it is hard.
>
> For those who neither have PD nor care for someone with it but

labor under the illusion that you are bulletproof, I hope that someone will be there for you when your illusions are stripped away and life in all its glorious mystery and wonder is finally revealed. (130)

Most of the dozens of lodestones that George Johnston publishes in The Unexpected Journey have no direct or obvious bearing on Parkinson's, but they are worth reading anyhow. Here are a few of my favorites:

It is better to struggle happily than to succeed miserably. (22)

Telling the truth never cost anyone a true friend. (40)

Exercise, if for no other reason than so that you can eat real butter. (46)

Strive to distinguish between subjective needs and objective necessities. (53)

In life's race, no one sprints across the finish line. (61)

In the end, all that wealth really provides is a more comfortable room to die in. (78)

He who dies with the most toys dies.
He who dies with no toys dies.
What is the real issue here? (80)

Always reach down to help pull someone up.
Never reach up to pull someone down. (116)

B13. *I Have Parkinson's: What Should I Do?*, by Ann Andrews. Laguna Beach, California: Basic Health Publications, 2011. xii + 179 pp.

> "I wish well-meaning friends and strangers, those without Parkinson's, wouldn't say they'd just heard of a cure."

The subtitle of *I Have Parkinson's: What Should I Do?* invites silly answers: Sit down and cry. Quick go out and buy long-term medical insurance. Buy a shotgun. Get your affairs in order (if you are having some). Punt (if you can still move your kicking foot). Get ready to shuffle off your mortal coil (whatever that is). Join the Catholic church. Write a book about what it is like to have Parkinson's. That last option seems to occur to increasing numbers of us.

There is a certain sameness to many of the books that get written by people with Parkinson's. They generally move from anger, denial, and fear to acceptance, optimism, and gratitude. They generally have chapters on symptoms, diagnosis, early-onset Parkinson's, finding a neurologist, medication options, surgical options, who to tell you have Parkinson's and when to tell them, what the disease does to marriages, families, and friendships, the importance of support groups, the importance of exercise, dietary considerations, appreciating the needs of your caregiver, and so on. The authors often describe their book as the one they wish they had had when they were first diagnosed. *I Have Parkinson's* is close enough to that standard pattern. Ann Andrews, a New Zealander diagnosed with Parkinson's in her fifties, begins her introduction thus:

> This book is written for people like me who have Parkinson's disease, and for our families, friends, doctors, and those working in the field. It began as a wish to share everything I've learned about Parkinson's since diagnosis nearly twelve years ago. It is still the book I wish I'd had when first diagnosed, though now it contains information that you might not need till later. (1)

She talks about how, when first diagnosed, she searched the Internet and found that the information available there tended to be "gloomy and depressing." She discovered that her growing list of friends with Parkinson's had had similar experiences. She enlisted their help in providing an alternative source of information: "We would like to share some of our knowledge and experience, and to provide something more individual, less clinical, and hopefully more reassuring than what we first read" (1).

The book is mostly about Ann Andrews's own experiences. It is appropriately personal. In her chapter on "Primary Symptoms and Diagnosis," for example, she describes the time when she was in the hospital for some initial testing:

> I was in a ward with six women, all much older than me. Four of us were patients of the same neurologist. One morning he came into the ward with two medical students and discussed the other women individually quite loudly, as if they were not present. The women were in the latter stages of Parkinson's and I found it immensely sad and depressing to see them treated with such disrespect. (15–16)

She also quotes in that chapter from the experiences of four others, Warwick, Clare, Kathy, and Michael. Here is an excerpt from Michael's reaction to his diagnosis:

> How was I to accept that life will never be the same? [...] Will I become dependent on my wife to care for me? And how will she deal with this change? Deep down inside me I know I cannot reverse this path and I am scared. Yes, I am scared in every sense of the word; scared that I may not be able to fend for myself, that I will have to be fed, toileted, and washed, and I have to accept that this is the way it's going to be. (21–22)

That kind of honesty about what it is like to have Parkinson's disease characterizes the book as a whole. Here is Ann Andrews on the term "caregiver," a term "probably conceived by a social worker reluctant to use the expression 'unpaid servant.' [...] If this sounds cynical, it's because the word 'caregiver' scares me so much I didn't want to use it in this book. It means someone who cares for another who can no longer care for themselves" (30–31).

In her closing chapter, "Getting On with Parkinson's," Ann Andrews resists the temptation to pretend that the later stages of the disease are a ton of fun: "I have to say that as time has gone on, I have lost confidence. There are days when I do feel feeble and irrelevant. I can't think quickly, my voice is quiet; I shake too much, and feel I have entirely lost my social skills. The more I feel like this, the more reduced I become" (157–58). Reading that we may feel the urge to try to give her hope that a cure will come, and come in time to make her well. She knows that is not going to happen. Her job is not to deny the reality or the seriousness of Parkinson's by saying it will soon disappear, but rather to get on with her life *with* Parkinson's:

> I wish well-meaning friends and strangers, those without Parkinson's, wouldn't say they'd just heard of a cure. When people first learn that you have Parkinson's, they often say things like: "I read somewhere recently that they've discovered a new drug" or "They're implanting stem cells now, aren't they?" [...] Getting on with life is what it's about, and that means getting on with Parkinson's. (160)

B14. *Living Well, Running Hard: Lessons Learned from Living with Parkinson's Disease* (second edition), by John Ball. Bloomington, Indiana: Universe, 2011. xii + 193 pp.

> "I learned quite late in life that no matter how well we think we're handling our individual challenges, none of us is really flying solo."

John Ball majored in English at the University of Washington, joined the Navy and was sent to Vietnam where he encountered Agent Orange. He returned and received his master's degree in English from California State University, Los Angeles. Then he almost finished his PhD in English literature at the University of California, Irvine, but never got around to finishing his doctoral dissertation on John Milton. Instead, he went to work for Honda of America. He played for some years on the Honda corporate softball team, but found himself growing more and more uncoordinated. He could rarely manage to hit the ball, could barely stumble to first base when he did, was a rotten catcher, and couldn't throw the ball back to the pitcher without at least one bounce. He sought the advice of several doctors about what had ailed him for the past dozen years, only to receive one misdiagnosis after another. Finally, just before John Ball turned forty, a doctor told him to try a little yellow pill called Sinemet. He did so and, much to the amazement of his softball team, he started playing softball amazingly well.

By then John Ball was married to a woman named Edna, whose mother had Parkinson's. Ball was delighted finally to have his disease identified as Parkinson's disease and to have a medicine that relieved some of his symptoms and let him move again with something like his old verve. He soon picked up again his old love of running, and a decade later, at age fifty-one, he ran his first full marathon—a feat he was to repeat some twenty-five more times in the coming years. At the urging of his neurologist he wrote about how he trained for and ran that first marathon. That essay caused him to be invited to talk to several Parkinson's support groups. That was his first experience with support groups. Before long he retired from his job at Honda and began working as an advocate for Parkinson's disease and helping to raise research dollars for several Parkinson's foundations. He became especially interested in the curative possibilities of stem cell research, though he was realistic about even that: "I think a real cure is unlikely in my lifetime, but not impossible" (180).

The subtitle of *Living Well, Running Hard* is *Lessons Learned from Living with Parkinson's Disease*. What are some of those lessons?

You can't always trust doctors. He went to several doctors before, a dozen years into the disease, he found one who got it right.

Keep everything in balance. The key to successful running is "keeping everything in balance, whether you have Parkinson's or not. For each of us, life is a constant balancing act; we try to keep personal needs, fitness, work, and family activities in the right proportions to ensure our mental and physical health" (52).

You can do more than you think you can, like run your first marathon when you've had Parkinson's for nearly twenty years.

Your Parkinson's affects not only you but others. "One of the cruelest aspects of Parkinson's is the suffering it inflicts on those who love and care for the person living with the disease; the caregivers may struggle with grief or a sense of helplessness or loss even more than the person they're caring for" (76).

Avoid the Parkinson's trap. "No matter how much I love my family, I sometimes put myself at risk just to show the world I'm still in control—even if I'm not. I don't want to be drawn into the Parkinson's trap, baited with temptations to 'give up.' When a doctor tells a patient, 'You have Parkinson's disease. It is degenerative, and there is no cure,' it would be easy to give up control to the doctor, or to family members, or to emptiness, anger, or despair. I don't think that's in anyone's best interest" (77).

Watch out for depression. If you begin to feel oppressed or isolated by your Parkinson's, you should seek help: "When I began thinking about suicide around October of 1997, I knew I was near the edge. Just driving down the street, I would feel a sudden powerful urge to drift left, into the oncoming traffic. […] With Edna's help, I finally admitted I needed professional care, so I went to see a therapist" (86–87).

Don't generalize. "I guess I thought of myself as a minor celebrity in the Parkinson's community and thought I had something important to share with them. But I soon learned each experience is unique. What works for me may have limited value to someone else. It would be a mistake to generalize from my experience any set of rules on how to deal with PD" (79). But he does his share of generalizing anyhow, especially in Chapter 23, "Blinding Flashes of the Obvious": "Listen to your doctors, your family, and your friends, but decide for yourself what you can or cannot do. […] Life gets more enjoyable when you stop worrying about what you can't do and focus on what you can do. […] If you think something is impossible, it is, until somebody else does it. […] Strength and fitness can overcome lots of challenges" (181–84).

That is all good advice, no doubt, but sometimes John Ball gives us reason to think that he believes his path is the right one, and that if he can make himself strong enough and fit enough to run some twenty years after his diagnosis, we should be able to do so also. That kind of thinking is dangerous. If we try it, we may hurt ourselves. If we don't try it we may feel as if we *should.*

B15. *Reverse Parkinson's Disease,* by John Pepper. Pittsburgh, Pennsylvania: Rosedog Books, 2011. 193 pp.

> "It is not my intention to falsely raise hopes by leading you to believe that my PD is cured."

John Pepper is one of us. Maybe.

Diagnosed in 1992, John Pepper had had almost twenty years of experience with Parkinson's by the time he published *Reverse Parkinson's Disease* in 2011. He speaks, then, with a certain authority when he describes the success of his treatment program. That program has three branches, one physical (exercise, diet), one mental (attitude, stress management), one chemical (he recommends an MAO-B inhibitor). It is difficult to argue with the first two of those. The third one is problematical.

In the end, the book does not fulfill the promise of its title. Readers who pick up *Reverse Parkinson's Disease* expecting to find a way to reverse or cure Parkinson's disease will probably be disappointed.

Shortly after his diagnosis, John Pepper quit his job as director of a South African printing business and began working to defeat Parkinson's and to share his story with others: "By sharing my experiences with other sufferers, especially those in the early stages of PD, I hope to help improve their quality of life, by restoring their self-confidence and giving them a better understanding of PD from a fellow sufferer's viewpoint" (12).

John Pepper's advice about the importance of physical exercise is strongly reinforced by virtually all people with Parkinson's and by their doctors. He is especially good on the importance of walking and walking *correctly*. Also useful is his advice about the importance of a positive mental attitude, of embracing optimism, and of exercising the brain.

The weakest part of *Reverse Parkinson's Disease* is the section on medications. John Pepper is not a doctor: "I don't pretend to have studied anything about the brain, or how it works" (92). His own physician told him to take one medicine and one only: the MAO-B inhibitor called Eldepryl. He references a research study that seemed to indicate that the drug could help people with Parkinson's. Here is his somewhat hedged conclusion: "I would personally assume that if taking Eldepryl could possibly slow down the progression of PD, then Eldepryl must have been one of the reasons why my PD started to improve" (66).

Particularly questionable is John Pepper's denigration of levodopa, the drug that most neurologists and most people with Parkinson's see as the gold standard of medications for this disease: "After taking Sinemet [a trade name for one form of levodopa] for three months I did not feel any benefit whatsoever. My movement problems had already been solved and the tremor had already disappeared. Sinemet does not mask all of the symptoms of PD but, those symptoms, which it does not mask, I was already able to overcome, by using my conscious brain" (66–67). John Pepper goes on to say that "levodopa medication should be a *last resort medication*, when all other PD medication has failed. [...] As a PD patient I personally think that early prescription of levodopa medication is irresponsible. That is just my opinion" (67).

We leave John Pepper's personal-experience-based ruminations on Parkinson's medications right there: they are just his opinion. We all have somewhat unique reactions to specific medications, and we recognize them as such. Unlike John Pepper, most of us are careful not to generalize.

In telling his story, John Pepper himself seems to step away from the promise of his title: "My gift of improved health is an exciting story and it needs to be told to the whole world, so that others will know what can happen, if we don't give up, when things go wrong. It is not my intention to falsely raise hopes by leading you to believe that my PD is cured. I still have most of the symptoms, but they are mostly under control and at a much lower level than they were in 1992" (13).

One of the most puzzling features of the book is that at the same time John Pepper wants us to believe that he is far better off after twenty years with Parkinson's than he was at the start, he also wants us to believe that he still has the symptoms. Indeed, he lists no fewer than thirty-five symptoms of Parkinson's that he still has: "1. Bad muscle co-ordination. 2. Constipation. 3. Choking and swallowing problems. 4. Rigidity. [...] 34. Confusion with which is the right and left side. 35. My calves become flexed when sitting" (101–02). That list of symptoms does not sound like the list one would have associated with a man who claims that his methods reduce or reverse the disease. (Readers who want another perspective on John Pepper's claims may want to have a look at my review of Norman Doidge (number A23 above).

Halfway through his book Pepper drops a little bombshell: that he may not have had Parkinson's at all. He reports that he went to a new neurologist, one who had never seen him before. After examining him the neurologist said to him, "You exhibit no symptoms of PD, and it is quite obvious that you never had it in the first place. You had what is known as Parkinsonism, which could have been caused by medication or by another chemical source, possibly crop spraying chemicals" (103). John Pepper rejects that diagnosis: "he never asked me what my existing symptoms were, or what I had had in the past" (103). John Pepper even hints that the neurologist in question had self-serving reasons for not wanting to investigate the possibility that anyone could reverse the progression of Parkinson's: "The only conclusion I can come to, is that I present a threat to the medical profession. If all his PD patients got to a stage, where they no longer need medication, nor need a neurologist any more, then I can understand his fears" (104). Serious charges, those.

In the end, John Pepper backs off: "On reflection, I realize that it does not really matter whether I do or don't have PD. It is purely academic" (111). But to those who might consider taking his advice about avoiding levodopa and taking an MAO-B inhibitor, it is not purely academic. It might be life or death.

We come away from *Reverse Parkinson's Disease* admiring its author's spirit and determination, but unconvinced that his experience is fully relevant to ours. If he never had Parkinson's to begin with, there was nothing to reverse. Until we know for sure, it is best to take this Pepper with a grain of salt.

B16. *Forty Thousand to One,* by Ben Petrick. Copyright 2011 KMP Enterprises. v + 177 pp.

> "I can remember standing on second base after my first hit (an RBI double) and looking up at 40,000 fans. [...] Almost exactly eight years later, my audience had gone from 40,000 to one."

What in the world is that title supposed to mean? Ben Petrick gives half of the answer on page 5: "The title of this book, *40,000 to One*, has two meanings. First, Americans have a one-in-40,000 chance of being stricken with Parkinson's disease. The second meaning, which is more personal, is revealed later in the book."

Ben Petrick, of Hillsboro, Oregon, showed brilliant promise as a professional baseball player. He was given a signing bonus of $495,000 when, right after high school in 1995, at age eighteen, he was recruited by the Colorado Rockies. After four brilliant years in the farm club, he was called up to the majors:

> My first at bat came in the second inning with Helton at second. The pitcher was Pirates ace Jason Schmidt. I ran the count to 3-and-1, got the fastball I was sitting on, and lined it into the gap for an RBI double. I cruised into second base standing up. Forty thousand fans stood and cheered. That wall of sound was so dense I could've hung a picture on it. (63–64)

A couple of months later, Ben Petrick began to notice that his body was not working quite right. His left hand had a slight tremor and his left toes cramped up when he took long jogs. He noticed that as catcher, when he held his glove out to give the pitcher a target, the glove shook. About that time his father Vern, then just fifty, told Ben that he had been diagnosed with Parkinson's disease. Ben already knew a little about Parkinson's because his grandfather—his mother's father—had the disease.

Ben Petrick suspected the worst. Several doctors, however, told him that he was too young to have Parkinson's. A doctor in Tucson told him that he had benign essential tremor. Finally he went to see a movement disorder specialist in Denver. This doctor diagnosed "Parkinsonism," and told him that if his symptoms got worse, "then you likely have Parkinson's disease" (26). The doctor wrote him a prescription for Requip. That diagnosis came just seven months after his father got his diagnosis. Ben Petrick found that the Requip helped him to play much better baseball—for a while. Two years later he went to the neurologist again. The doctor took him off Requip and put him on Sinemet. Ben Petrick found that the new medication helped him to play much better baseball—for a while. "By 2003," he says, "my medication intake has become absolutely reckless. I keep my pills in my right pocket, because if I go 'off'—meaning my medication ceases to work sooner than I expect—I won't be able to use my left hand to get them out" (31–32).

He knew that, despite his heavy doses of Sinemet, he was not playing well: "My swing was funky, and at the plate I was making adjustments to my adjustments. I was constantly hooking the ball foul. Catching was a near impossibility, so I was now almost exclusively an outfielder" (82).

Disappointed in his performance, the Colorado Rockies traded Ben Petrick to the Detroit Tigers, but his decline continued: "I'm tired of hiding, tired of taking pills, tired of poor performances. I collect no hits in my first ten at bats, with seven strikeouts, and the Tigers released me. I feel sweet,

sweet relief" (32). Not long after, in 2004, at age twenty-seven, Ben Petrick announced that he had been diagnosed with Parkinson's disease and was retiring from baseball. He went back to Hillsboro and worked for a while as a coach.

He married his girlfriend Kellie and they had a daughter Makena. But his disease got worse and soon he had to give up coaching, go on disability, and take care of his daughter so his wife could go back to work teaching third grade. He and Kellie moved across the street from his parents' house in Hillsboro so his mother could help care for his daughter when he was "off." But his illness was tearing him apart:

> Every time Kellie enters a room, I want to ask, "Wouldn't you be happier with someone else?" But I don't ask. I don't want to know the answer. I'm overcome by a sadness that seems to be the very definition of the word: to look at a woman and a child, and love them madly, desperately, deeply—and at the same time think I'm hurting them with my very presence. This is where the heartbreak starts. [...] I've gone from playing in front of 40,000 screaming fans to an audience of one. And she needs her dad. (37–38)

As he put it later in the book, referring to his recollection of that wonderful day in September 1999, when he got his first major-league hit: "I can remember standing on second base after my first hit (an RBI double) and looking up at 40,000 fans giving a standing ovation" (101). Then he adds, "almost exactly eight years later, my audience had gone from 40,000 to one" (102). And that is the second and "more personal" explanation of the title, *40,000 to One*.

There is more to Ben Petrick's story. There is his account of his team's reaction to the events of 9/11/2001 (75ff). There is his disastrous first deep brain stimulation (DBS) surgery that not only failed but almost killed him, and a while later, his second DBS surgery that was more successful (110ff).

How can readers of this repetitious book with the strange title connect with a baseball player who exits early? Well, who of us will not resonate with comments like this: "Parkinson's comes with emotional issues that land heavily, even on its most tenacious sufferers: embarrassment when holding up the line at the store while fumbling for your wallet. Self-consciousness as you watch your loved ones watch you, as you tread cautiously around a home now riddled with booby traps. Fear on top of fear that you'll slip irreversibly into dementia" (88).

B17. *Parkinson's Dreams about Me: My Dance with the Shaking Palsy*, **by Rick Herman. Copyright Rick Herman, 2012. 183 pp.**

> "One of the most difficult things about having Parkinson's disease, which seems as true to me now as it did six or seven years ago, is that it takes away capabilities I've always considered fundamental to my identity."

Rick Herman was an avid singer, guitar-player, songwriter, editor, and bicycling enthusiast. His only major problem was persistent depression. Then he developed a second major problem. While biking to work one day he was struck by an automobile. Not long after the accident he was diagnosed, at about age forty, with Parkinson's disease.

He wondered whether the accident somehow triggered the disease, but there was no way to be sure. He also wondered if there was a causal connection between his depression and his Parkinson's but, again, there was no way to be sure. He continued for several years to work in the publishing and the music industries, but before long his symptoms got worse. People began to notice the shaking and lurching as well as the difficulty he had strumming his guitar. He himself began to notice the difficulty he had processing information at work. He had trouble making plans, putting bits of information into their place in a coherent whole. He decided to work half-time, but found the going too hard, too exhausting, and too frustrating. He finally quit his job altogether. And there he was, aged fifty, officially disabled, and more depressed than ever. He tried deep brain stimulation, but the results were at best minimal. Now what?

Rick Hermann decided to write a book about his experience with Parkinson's. In twenty-five short essay-chapters he tells us, in language honest, eloquent, and cynical, what it has been like. It is not a pretty picture:

> I am certain that if there is a "cures Parkinson's" pill, the list of side-effects and contra-indications would look something like this: "Caution, this medication may cause liver damage, hypertension, hallucinations, suicidal thoughts, vascular parkinsonism, and death." (26)

One of the cardinal symptoms of Parkinson's disease is

bradykinesia, a fancy way of saying that PWPs move like tortoises on terra firma. Slowly. Parkinson's is not a condition that is defined only by rhythmic tremor or uncontrollable dyskinesia. Parkinson's disease, in fact, is the progressive loss of the ability to move at all. (27)

I get discouraged that I literally have to relearn how to walk every morning. (30)

A sexual relationship for those with chronic illness of any kind requires flexibility and innovation. But, for anyone, physical limitations and drug side-effects, as well as coexisting conditions such as depression, can turn love-making into a difficult and frustrating experience. This can be due to both disease progression and the side-effects of Parkinson's medications on one's libido. (43)

In general, when people tell me I look "good," they are being incredibly thoughtful and trying to help. But all I can think is, why do I look so good if I'm feeling so crummy? (54)

One of the most difficult things about having Parkinson's disease, which seems as true to me now as it did six or seven years ago, is that it takes away capabilities I've always considered fundamental to my identity. (73)

In late 2001 I was complaining to my neurologist about my work situation. I had cut back to four hours a day because of crushing fatigue and cognitive changes. The rest of the time I spent either girding up for or recovering from those four hours. (80)

His neurologist's response to that last negative lament is interesting: "Today is as good as you're ever going to feel." Not much room for optimism in that pronouncement, is there? But his neurologist went on to give him positive advice: "Think about how you want to use your time and energy for the rest of your life" (80). That may be good advice for all of us. Is it not better for us to face squarely the fundamental fact of our disease: that it only gets worse, never better? Is it not better for us to think about how to make the best of the years and powers that we have left rather than waste those years and powers lamenting the fact that we do not have more years and more powers?

What are we to make of the title of Rick Hermann's book, *Parkinson's Dreams about Me?* So far as I can tell, he means by that title to signal his empty powerlessness in the face of his disease: "I don't dream about Parkinson's disease. Sometimes I think that Parkinson's disease dreams about me. Maybe even dreams me into existence, making me confront my shadow self" (26). It is sad to think that Rick Hermann has come to believe that he exists only as the impotent dream-eunuch of a debilitating disease. It is sad to think that he believes that "with Parkinson disease there is always an hourglass whose sand is about to run out" (120). The book is of course not all negative and cynical, but even the hope he expresses seems often to come out sounding like despair: "Then one morning I wake up and it doesn't feel so bad, so complicated, so hopeless. I feel the stirrings of possibility. I take a deep breath, and I try again (and again) to lead the life I've been given" (136).

B18. *Parkinson's Humor: Funny Stories about My Life with Parkinson's Disease*, by Beverly Ribaudo. Copyright 2012 by Beverly Ribaudo. 214 pp.

> "We hate it when people feel sorry for us. Being blind is normal for her and being a Parkie is now normal for me, so please help us get up if we fall down, but don't feel sorry for us."

Yuma Bev tells the story about the day her Wonderful Husband was out jeeping with the neighbors near their home in Yuma, Arizona. She was home alone and saw on the television a commercial showing an inviting-looking bubble bath. She was feeling "stiff and achy (a normal occurrence for me)," so she decided to try a bubble bath herself. "Ahhhh, it felt sooo good. I could feel myself relaxing and all the stiffness melting away. It was absolutely enjoyable." But then the water cooled and she found herself trapped in the tub: "There was nothing to grab a hold of to pull myself up. The towel bar was too far away. The sides of the tub were slick fiberglass. There was a small grab bar but it was on my 'wrong' side and only about ten inches above the tub. There I was, stuck in the tub. The cell phone was out on the kitchen counter. The neighbors on both sides were out somewhere in the desert with my Wonderful Husband. HELP!" (32–33). She finally managed to wiggle herself around so she was facing in the other direction, took hold of the grab bar with her good hand, steadied herself with the other hand on the spigot, and managed to climb out of the tub.

What is the point of the story? Is it that we should pity people with Parkinson's for the agonies and dangers they face? Is it a lesson about the foolishness of people with Parkinson's taking bubble baths when home alone with no cell phone nearby? Is it about the need to make one's home safer by installing extra hand rails and grab bars? Is it a lesson about how her not-so-Wonderful Husband should have been more careful about leaving his Parkinson's wife alone for so long? For Yuma Bev it is none of those things: "By the time my Wonderful Husband and the neighbors came home, I was fine and had turned my misadventure into a funny story to be shared over pizza, even joking about the group of handsome firemen coming to my rescue. That's just me; I find humor anywhere I can" (33).

Parkinson's Humor began as the blog of a woman who took the chat-room name "Yuma Bev." Most of the one-hundred-plus stories are very short. The one above, entitled "Rub a Dub-Dub," is less than two pages long. Most are shorter than that and, in some, the humor seems forced. There is "David and Me," the story about her older brother:

> Mom had pneumonia during her pregnancy and David got the mumps and measles when he was just weeks old. My grandmother didn't pay attention when she was changing his diaper and he rolled off the table. He fell (or got pushed) off a two-story building, fell off a motorcycle, got severe burns on his feet, and got hit by a car. When Mom was seven months pregnant with me, she was told David was retarded. [...] The doctors told Mom to put David in an institution, but she said NO, he belonged at home. (155)

Where is the humor in that story? Well, Yuma Bev says she learned to laugh from her retarded older brother: "David was always happy, laughing or smiling. [...] I have a special place in my heart for anyone who is different, and my Parkinson's seems minor compared to David's life. I taught David how to tie his shoes and pee like a man, but he taught me how to LIVE and LOVE and most of all . . . LAUGH!" (156–57).

One of the most charming features of *Parkinson's Humor* is Yuma Bev's penchant for writing lyrics. Here is the first of twelve stanzas of a song she calls "My Dopamine":

> There's a drug called dopamine
> It helps me thru my daily routine

> Without it I might cause a scene
> I gotta take my dopamine (116)

Another engaging feature of Yuma Bev's book is her on-line friendship with a young blind woman named Cat. She has never met Cat face-to-face, but they are Twitter friends. In "What a Cat Taught a Parkie," she tells how she communicates with her friend who lives far away in West Virginia:

> She uses screen-reader software designed for the blind to "read' what is on the screen. Twitter is her main connection to the outside and she "talks" to people around the world. She is curious, smart, sympathetic, and fun, plus she has a great sense of humor. [...] She likes to help people as well. When she saw a post about how my fingers stutter when I type, she came up with some great suggestions for Parkinson's people who have trouble typing. (114)

In "How Do I Describe a Fox to a Cat," Yuma Bev says,

> Despite the fact that I am old enough to be her Mom and we live on opposite sides of the country and I have Parkinson's and she is blind, we have much in common. We hate it when people feel sorry for us. Being blind is normal for her and being a Parkie is now normal for me, so please help us get up if we fall down, but don't feel sorry for us. (101)

I come away from *Parkinson's Humor* admiring Yuma Bev's spirit and courage in the face of her Parkinson's. If some of the humor seems forced, is not a forced humor better than self-pity, blame, or bitterness? She has plenty to feel bitter about. Her grandmother and her father both had Parkinson's. Her mother died slowly of lung cancer. Her brother was retarded. Her first husband died in a fiery car crash when she was twenty-three. She herself has a particularly painful kind of Parkinson's. If anyone has a right to feel that life has dealt her a rotten hand, she does, but she does not complain. If anyone deserves to be pitied she does, yet she rejects our pity. What is the secret of her good cheer? "That's just me; I find humor anywhere I can" (33).

B19. *A Soft Voice in a Noisy World: A Guide to Dealing and Healing with Parkinson's Disease,* by Karl A. Robb. Fairfax, Virginia: RobbWorks, 2012. xx + 303 pp.

> "Through Reiki, along with massage, yoga, mild exercise, a hopeful attitude, and a vegetarian diet, I have held steady and reduced my dosage of medication, rather than needing to ramp it up as is expected in Parkinson's disease."

Karl Robb was only seventeen when he first noticed that something was wrong with his body. He became less flexible. He slouched in his chair. His feet started shuffling and dragging. His shoes wore out at different rates. When he walked his arms did not swing. Six years later, after visiting many doctors, he finally got at age twenty-three what turned out to be an accurate diagnosis: young-onset Parkinson's disease. When he found out, he searched for some sort of manual that would tell him about the disease and how to react effectively to the diagnosis. He could find nothing. Eventually he decided to write for others the book he wished he had been able to find then. *A Soft Voice in a Noisy World* is that book.

The book has fifty-nine chapters divided into five parts. In Part One, entitled If Doctors Had All the Answers, Medicine Wouldn't Be Called a "Practice," Karl Robb gives vent to some of the frustrations he has known as a not-very-patient patient. The tone of the section is revealed in his invitation to his readers to take "The Pledge of the Ill":

> I am worthy of being cared for by medical practitioners who treat me with respect and are willing to listen to me. I deserve to be recognized by my physician or other healthcare provider as a person with a life, not just as someone with a medical problem and a chart. My physician owes me the understanding to speak with me as an equal and as a human being. (7)

The titles of some of the chapters in Part One reveal the author's annoyance with doctors. For example: 3, "Frustration with Doctors"; 4, "Finding the Right New Doctor"; 5, "Is Your Current Doctor Satisfactory?"; 6, "Getting a Second Opinion"; and 9, "How to Talk to Doctors." Chapter 9 ends with a one-page "Challenge to Doctors" with advice like this: "Refrain from treating me like a number. [...] Remember my name. [...] Really observe me and listen to what I say" (68).

In Part Two, *Living with Parkinson's*, the author continues to voice his frustration. Even many of the positive things that he says about the disease come off sounding negative: "Everyone has flaws in body, mind, or character, and disease may help us to address these imperfections. With time and effort, this can become your opportunity to learn from the humility that comes with disease" (75). Again, the chapter titles tell the story: 12, "This Disease Isn't Fair"; 13, "Dealing with Depression"; 16, "Structure Your Life to Gain Some Control"; 18, "Two-Headed Monster"; 19, "Sickness Happens"; and 21, "Voice."

I should say something about Chapter 21, "Voice," if only because the issue of voice provides the title of *A Soft Voice in a Noisy World*. The author's negativity is familiar by now:

> There is no getting around the fact that we're judged by our ability to communicate verbally. Many good ideas and thoughts from someone with speech difficulties are not always heard or recognized due to a lack of patience or willingness on the part of the listener to let these ideas and thoughts be expressed fully. (111)

It is well known that a gradually weakening voice often comes along with Parkinson's disease: "Whether someone's voice is soft and muted or broken and barely intelligible, if the listener makes a judgment or loses interest in what is being said, then the content will be missed" (112). One solution, Karl Robb says, is for people with Parkinson's to stay away from "noisy places" (112).

Chapter 25, "PD Defined," seems straightforward enough, until we read the alternative negative definitions that the author offers: "Parkinson's is expecting reliability from your body and mind, and often getting cooperation from neither. [...] Parkinson's is a python-like lead shell that slowly encases your feet and the rest of your body. [...] Parkinson's is a thief that may slowly steal your independence" (125–26).

Part Three, *Support Groups and Relationships*, is my favorite part. It starts off with the negativity we have come to expect from Karl Robb:

> For the majority of my years with Parkinson's disease, I was anti-support group. My reasoning (or lack thereof) came from my few sporadic encounters with peer groups in which participants were completely focused on their problems. Many seemed to prefer

complaining to helping each other explore solutions. Some patients and care partners in those groups obviously wanted to vent their frustration at being at the mercy of Parkinson's disease, robbed of their freedom of movement and voice. (157)

In other words, Karl Robb was as impatient with the whining negativity of others with Parkinson's as I may have been with his. Then he attended a few more support groups, even started one of his own, and changed his view: "My misconception that attending a support group was a sign of weakness, depressing, a waste of time, and a big pity-party was permanently erased" (158–59). A good support group, he says, can provide information, comradeship, a chance to laugh, a chance to help others, and the comfort of knowing that we are not alone with our disease.

In Part Four, *Reiki, Meditation, and Other Complementary Therapies*, Karl Robb attempts to broaden the base of our knowledge about Parkinson's disease. He suggests that instead of relying only on Western-style medication and surgery, we should give careful consideration to complementary therapies like Reiki, qigong, yoga, meditation, visualization, exercise, and massage. He is particularly skeptical of deep brain stimulation (DBS), in part because it is invasive and risky. He acknowledges that it seems to have helped many patients, but is troubled by the fact that no one knows how or why DBS works, when it does work.

The same argument, of course, could be made about Reiki, a Japanese meditational treatment that Karl Robb has tried with what he claims is great success. He defines Reiki as "the transferring of the universal energy that is all around us to renew the depletion of our energy" (193). He claims that "through Reiki, along with massage, yoga, mild exercise, a hopeful attitude, and a vegetarian diet, I have held steady and reduced my dosage of medication, rather than needing to ramp it up as is expected in Parkinson's disease. The proof is in the results!" (230). Many readers will question his use of the word "proof." He claims, further that he is "amazed and overjoyed that I have had the ability to consistently improve and show real signs of getting better" (234). "Today," he continues, "I can say that I am better now than I was ten years ago. Having had Parkinson's for over twenty years, I see this as remarkable and nearly miraculous" (242).

At the start of his book, the author says, "If you get only one thing out of this book, in my view, it should be the understanding that you have more power and control over your well-being than you know. From your choice of the drugs you take, to the food you eat and the doctors who advise your progress, you are in charge" (5).

In Part Five, *Raising Awareness and Effecting Change*, Karl Robb argues that people with Parkinson's should strive to educate the public—"our communities, the government, and yes, even doctors, about Parkinson's disease" (249). The idea that lay people have the knowledge and the obligation to educate doctors will, of course puzzle some patients and most doctors.

B20. *The Peripatetic Pursuit of Parkinson Disease*, by NeuroWriters. Little Rock, Arkansas: Parkinson's Creative Collective, 2013. 319 pp.

> "It's like you get up in the morning and think, I'd like to do this and that today, but first I have to check with the board of directors, and Mr. Parkinson is the Chairman of the Board."

It is always good to hear about Parkinson's from the people who know it best—the men and women who have the disease. *The Peripatetic Pursuit of Parkinson Disease* gives us a welcome window into the lives and thoughts of a wide variety of such people.

Who wrote this book? The title page lists eleven specific authors, in alphabetical order, and mentions many unnamed "contributors from the international Parkinson community." On page 6 we find the photographs of those eleven, plus the photographs and first names of two more. No leader or editor-in-chief is singled out. Instead we find the statement that "we made decisions by consensus, worked in harmony." Separated by distance, they worked in Skype meetings to bring the work of many individuals with Parkinson's together in this book. The Foreword is by John M. Grohol, PsyD, the founder of an online community known as NeuroTalk, but he was apparently not one of the writers or editors of *The Peripatetic Pursuit of Parkinson Disease*.

This imprecision about the editorial process can be explained in part by a desire to provide legal protection to the authors and publishers in case someone wanted to sue: "The reader assumes all responsibility and risk, if any, for the use of any of the general information found within the book" (2).

Can the information and the advice given in the book be trusted? The answer is that you will have to decide that for yourself. For example, in a section on "Helpful Hints for Parkinson Carers" we find this advice: "Discourage use of a cane (walking stick), walker, wheelchair, or power chair until absolutely necessary." If I follow that advice, walk out without my cane, fall and break a hip, can I sue? Probably not. No specific author of that advice is listed, and in any case, the legal disclaimer seems to leave me no recourse. Does my fall mean that the advice was bad? Perhaps, but perhaps not. Is it really bad advice to encourage a person with Parkinson's to try to manage as long as possible without depending on an assistive device? Would a cane have prevented my fall? Was my use of the cane "absolutely necessary"? (For what it is worth, I generally do not use a cane or walker at home, but do when I go out.)

The introduction states that "this book was written by people with Parkinson disease, for people with Parkinson disease, their families, their friends, and all who love and care for them" (9). The various chapters are variously useful.

Chapter 1, "Parkinson Basics," will be of particular interest to the newly diagnosed. It contains the brief narratives of a number of patients, gives lists of symptoms often associated with Parkinson's, lists of medications often prescribed and their possible side effects, shows what a number of people who have had deep brain stimulation (DBS) feel about whether it helped them, gives advice about how to react to the diagnosis and when to tell others about it, and lists the things people hate most about having Parkinson's. My favorite quotation from Chapter 1: "Parkinson doesn't kill you. But there are no survivors" (70).

Chapter 2, "More than a Movement Disorder," challenges the common assumption that Parkinson's is entirely or even mostly about motor disorders. For many patients, difficulties with movement are the least of their worries. Just as frightening are other problems that can come with the disease or with the medications prescribed for it: anxiety, apathy, confusion, constipation, delusions, dementia, depression, drooling, executive dysfunction, extreme fatigue, hallucinations, impulse control, incontinence, nausea, sexual dysfunctions, sleep problems, speech difficulties, weight loss or weight gain. My favorite quotation from Chapter 2: "It's like you get up in the morning and think, I'd like to do this and that today, but first I have to check with the board of directors, and Mr. Parkinson is the Chairman of the Board" (87).

Chapter 3, "Helping Ourselves," sings the praises of exercise—almost any exercise: biking, boxing, dancing, going to gyms and health clubs, hiking, paddling, pedaling, playing a musical instrument, rowing, sailing, singing, swimming, tai chi, walking, yoga. But there are other things we can do also: practice good nutrition, use spices like ginger, curcumin, and turmeric, filter our drinking water, meditate and get massages, stay active socially, laugh, stay engaged in life. My favorite quotation from Chapter 3: "If I do nothing, I get nothing, but then nothing is expected if I do nothing so at least I'm not disappointed in the results. However, I strive to push on, by realizing that too long of a hesitation is actually a stop, and too long a stop is actually a regression. It's like paddling a canoe upstream. Your effort, or lack of it, determines your direction" (124).

Chapter 4, "Quality of Life," is about ways to have more enjoyment despite the reality of a diagnosis of Parkinson's. It raises issues like coping in the workplace, making a good transition away from work, exercising the brain as well as the body, finding ways to enjoy what we have and finding new things to enjoy as the disease progresses, finding grace, coping alone and sharing the burden, finding alternative treatments, accepting life in the slow lane, and enjoying our children. My favorite quotation from Chapter 4: "Hey, these things happen . . . and I'm absolutely sure that my husband and daughter, as well as myself, have been made stronger by it" (157).

Chapter 5, "The Difficult Bits," deals with late-disease issues like home care, hospitals, nursing homes, living wills, advance directives, hospice, and dying. The chapter is prefaced with this advice: "You may wish to defer reading this chapter until you feel you need the information" (168). I am not sure that it is wise to delay thinking about end-stage Parkinson's. Refusing to think about such issues can be disastrous for both you and your family. My favorite quotation in Chapter 5: "It is not dying we are afraid of, it is dying badly" (201).

Chapters 6, "PD Activism," 7, "Advocacy in Action," and 8, "Going International," give advice about becoming an advocate for Parkinson's, becoming part of the wider medical, political, and advocacy movements by donating, going to walks, participating in on-line chat rooms, joining and supporting local, national, and international foundations, volunteering for medical research, and working to limit the use of certain chemicals and toxic substances in farming and military operations. My favorite quotation from Chapters 6–8: "Despite two hundred years of effort, we do not know the cause, the course, or the cure" (245).

The Peripatetic Pursuit of Parkinson Disease is a rich and valuable compendium of essays, reports, opinions, narratives, pleas, and poems by many different men and women who have Parkinson's. Its chief strength is that it presents the direct views of people who write with refreshing honesty about their own experiences with the disease. Its chief weakness is closely related to its chief strength: it remains a widely diverse collection of views. There is virtually no effort to bring the various views together into a consensus view.

The book lives up to its title, *The Peripatetic Pursuit of Parkinson Disease*. The authors tell us that the word "peripatetic" derives from the Greek word meaning "given to walking about." They remind us that a "peripatetic school" is an informal school and that Aristotle was given to lecturing while walking about. In this book "peripatetic" suggests not a wise Aristotle giving coherent lectures, but meandering teachers who all seem to stroll around and talk at the same time. There is much useful information in this book, but it might have profited from an Aristotle who would help us to separate the wisdom from the whining, the factual from the frivolous, the true from the merely heartfelt.

B21. *Reboot and Rejoice: How I Healed from Parkinson's Disease Using the Body/Mind Practice of Qigong*, by Bianca Mollé. Mettamorphix Press, 2013. viii + 144 pp.

> "It's all about vibration, and how every living thing vibrates in some way. We all want to raise our vibrational levels to feel better, and in so doing can often raise the vibrations of those round us."

Bianca Mollé loved her job as a middle school teacher, but by April of 2008, her physical tremors, pain, stiffness, and instability had become so bad that she consulted a neurologist. He diagnosed Parkinson's disease and prescribed Sinemet and Requip. The medicines helped some, but her symptoms forced her to request early retirement from the teaching job she had enjoyed for twenty-five years. Many of those symptoms—stiffness, pain, imbalance—persisted. Newly retired, she had the time to explore other ways of healing herself.

In June 2009, she attended a "Healer Within" workshop in California, where she tried qigong. She soon became convinced that it helped with her symptoms. When she learned about a three-week "Healing Intensive Retreat" scheduled that fall in Guilin, China, she signed up: "Needless to say, those around me were astonished. I barely knew qigong or the people who were teaching it, yet I was going to spend three weeks in Guilin, practicing and deeply learning qigong" (32).

To ready herself for that experience, she weaned herself from her Western-style medicines before leaving for China. The experience in China was life-altering for her. On her return home she continued to practice qigong two or three hours a day. Not long after that she went to her neurologist, who told her that she no longer presented Parkinson's symptoms: "And it's not just me, some people with Parkinson's in the qigong community are demonstrating steady signs of improvement—like reduced tremors, better balance, increased flexibility in shoulders, faster, more fluid walking, and more energy" (40–41).

Bianca Mollé began giving talks about her experience and helping others heal themselves through qigong:

> I am contacted regularly by a number of people with Parkinson's and some of them perplex me. They want to know if I really practiced for several hours a day because they don't have the time for that. It seems to me that all serious chronic conditions are screaming at us to pay attention and to devote positive time and energy to making ourselves well NOW before any further deterioration occurs. The "pay now or pay later" adage applies so well here. (55)

Bianca Mollé got a lot of attention for having apparently cured herself of Parkinson's just by stopping taking Western-style medication and starting Eastern-style meditation. She was happy to help others who came to her for help: "My mission is to encourage the undecided. If you're even contemplating my suggestion, you are listening to an inner voice that would serve you well in being further cultivated. 'Just Say Yes.' Now is the time for you to care for yourself, your primary obligation on this planet" (57–58). She is careful to offer appropriate legal disclaimers about her slender book: "*This was written for informational purposes only. It is not suggested medical advice for any individual. Content should not be considered medical advice. The writer is not a medical professional*" (65).

How can Parkinson's disease, which we are told is progressive, degenerative, and irreversible, respond so well to qigong? Bianca Mollé does not pretend to know the answer: "I must admit, I felt a bit like Harry Potter, bumbling about Hogwarts, being celebrated for something and not knowing the how or why of it, and sometimes embarrassed and/or confused by the praise and attention" (75). She speculates that the "inner self knows the answers and that the body reflects these truths. It's all about vibration, and how every living thing vibrates in some way. We all want to raise our vibrational levels to feel better, and in so doing can often raise the vibrations of those round us" (77). If you are confused by such statements, it may—or may not—make you feel better to realize that she is, too:

> I'm still basically a bonehead when it comes to the healing arts and the world of energy. But that's what restored my health and vitality, and I will work tirelessly to figure it out and explain it because I want others to be able to experience the happiness, health, and second chance at life that I currently enjoy. (77)

I am pleased to learn that Bianca Mollé is happy and healthy, but she has not convinced me that what worked for her will work for others.

Reboot and Rejoice closes with the information that Bianca Mollé has made a business of her convictions: "I have established a practice as a wellness coach and consultant, and have a client and reader base composed of people with Parkinson's and/or their families or caregivers, and of people with other chronic conditions" (90). I suppose, however, that most of us with Parkinson's would feel better about availing ourselves of her services if she were able to explain how qigong is helpful, how it works to cure the disease. We appreciate her modesty in proclaiming herself "a bonehead when it comes to the healing arts," but such modesty does not inspire confidence.

B22. *Both Sides Now: A Journey from Researcher to Patient*, by Alice Lazzarini, PhD. Copyright 2014 by Alice Lazzarini. xii + 213 pp.

> "And who will take care of me when I require assistance with daily living? My answer is, 'I really don't know.' But when it happens, I know I will be able to rely on the people around me to help me figure it out—people whom I've loved and who love me."

What I found most interesting in Alice Lazzarini's memoir is her account of her frustrating struggle to balance the conflicting demands made on her as the daughter of difficult parents, the wife of an unreliable husband, the mother of dependent children, the student of unsympathetic teachers, the employee of insensitive bosses, the researcher of underfunded science projects, the counselor of frightened patients, and finally the patient afflicted with a distressing disease. Life for Alice Lazzarini has been a struggle of unusual proportions, but she came through it all at peace with herself and her lot, proud of all that she accomplished.

She was particularly proud of the work she did as a genetics and family counselor to people stricken with Huntington's disease. She spends more time in her book talking about that dreadful disease and the havoc it wreaks on those unlucky enough to have it than she does talking about Parkinson's. She seemed to have little emotional connection to Parkinson's. When "the Boss," Roger Duvoisin, the man in charge of Columbia Presbyterian Parkinson's Clinic in New York, offered her a job helping investigate the possible genetic origins of Parkinson's disease, she was openly resistant. She found Parkinson's patients to be stiff, cautious, inhibited, and boring:

> "I prefer my fun-loving Huntington patients to those stiff 'Parkies'," I insisted. To me, the dance-like movements that one sees in Huntington patients represent a wonderfully free loss of inhibition and spontaneous behavior. The cautious rigidity seen in Parkinson's patients screamed, BORING. (111)

The title of *Both Sides Now* refers apparently to the fact that Alice Lazzarini knew Parkinson's disease first from the research "side" as someone who helped to trace the hereditary configuration of the disease back to the Contursi village in Italy. The other "side," then, was the patient side. She was diagnosed with Parkinson's at age sixty-three. It must be particularly difficult for people who are professionally knowledgeable about Parkinson's to find themselves suddenly served with the dreaded diagnosis. Alice Lazzarini seemed incapable of escaping the self-pity that is a common reaction to such a diagnosis. She referred to Parkinson's as a "death sentence" that brought on "the demise of a wonderful career" (143). She leapt immediately to what I call "futurizing"—imagining how awful it would be later when the "time bomb" exploded and left her immobile and dependent:

> Daybreak coaxes me awake. Once upon a time—before Parkinson's forced me to stop working—my first conscious thought was whether or not it was a work day. [...] Now when I wake, I am acutely aware that my time is always my own. I can plan every day at whatever pace is comfortable—crowding in many errands or relaxing with a book. But, I realize my right arm is shaking and I am

> not intentionally moving it. Then a new dawning, a different kind
> of awakening—a realization that the movements are a time bomb
> that is ticking away as my brain cells die. My time is my own now
> only until that bomb goes off, until I can no longer play with my
> grandchildren or drive to my nephew's karate tournament, until I can
> no longer move, no longer take care of myself. That is Parkinson's
> disease. Ten, twenty, one hundred times a day when my hand begins
> to shake uncontrollably, the reality dawns again. (27)

It never seems to occur to Alice Lazzarini that all people, whether or not
they have Parkinson's, face such a time bomb as they grow older. She never
seems to figure out that being born is itself a "death sentence" for all of
us. She seems unable to stop feeling sorry for herself as a woman unfairly
afflicted with a debilitating disease.

Realizing that she will one day be incapable of taking care of herself,
and that Bob, her husband of forty-odd years, will not be able to take good
care of her when that day comes, she ends her marriage and buys herself a
condo. Still she futurizes:

> And who will take care of me when I require assistance with daily
> living? My answer is, "I really don't know." But when it happens,
> I know I will be able to rely on the people around me to help me
> figure it out—people whom I've loved and who love me. (144)

Alice Lazzarini's *Both Sides Now* is less about Parkinson's disease
than about the distressed reactions of a woman who has trouble thinking
positively about her diagnosis. She can see in it only the decline and
dependence that will eventually make her life miserable. She mentions her
hope for a cure for Parkinson's, but her hope is not convincing:

> Because Parkinson's progresses slowly, one is faced with constantly
> confronting change—a new awareness with the loss of each piece
> of your former self. Pain and sorrow inevitably occur as the ability
> to do what once was easy, decreases. Pity parties are allowed. Give
> in and feel it. [...] And, because Parkinson's progresses slowly, you
> have every right to maintain the hope—as I do—that researchers
> will make further exponential progress in our lifetime. (164–65)

I am not so sure that others facing a diagnosis of Parkinson's will be well-
served by *Both Sides Now*.

B23. *Leading the Dance: Living Well with Parkinson's Disease*, **by Sel Kerans. Copyright Sel Kerans, 2014. 51 pp.**

> "Get out, Parkinson's. I have no room for you in my life! Go! Now!"

S el Kerans is an educator and photographer who lives in Queensland, Australia. He was diagnosed at age fifty. He describes the news as making him feel "like paddling a kayak downstream, unprepared for the dangerous rapids that suddenly appeared. [...] Hurtling through the rapids was no joy ride. I shouted in anger, held on, and tried not to panic through having my life tossed around and tipped over" (3). Later he refers to having Parkinson's as trying to avoid a train wreck (see 10–11). He soon drops both the nautical and railroad metaphors and shifts to a dance metaphor:

> Sharing a life with Parkinson's disease can be like having a necessary but uneasy relationship with an unwelcome intruder. It is important to find a way to get along with the intruder, whilst openly hoping to expel it one day. It becomes necessary to engage in a less-than-courtly dance with Parkinson's disease (the intruder) across a dance floor of life upheaval. [...] The aim is to make the connection, though unwelcome, and to learn as much as possible about how Parkinson's disease may present as a dance partner, in order to control the disease as the leader of the dance. [...] The choice can be yours. Your life can be your own, albeit for a time with the unwelcome intruder; that dance partner you must learn to lead and whom you may one day get to see off! (6)

Sel Kerans is an optimist. He thinks research scientists will one day soon find a cure for the disease. The job of people with Parkinson's is to keep our bodies as healthy as possible until that cure comes our way. Keeping our bodies healthy is easy enough. It is a matter of following six simple but important rules: eat wisely, stay away from alcohol, get enough sleep, exercise, avoid being alone by seeking out positive friends. Perhaps most important is to maintain a positive attitude:

> I believe in the power of the mind and positive suggestion; that both change and success come from belief, with a concerted and

continued effort in *willing it to be*—that the body has an incredible capacity to heal itself, starting with the right mindset and in accord with a complimentary, ongoing course of action. There is always hope. Never lose that. You have to be positive, convincing yourself daily that you can heal your body. (18)

One of Sel Kerans's specific suggestions is to imagine yourself riding joyously along in your car listening to your favorite music:

> You dance in your seat, and tap the steering wheel with one hand in time with the beat. Then in the joyous moments, you feel Parkinson's being drawn from your head and body by the buffeting breeze escaping through the window to the rushing air outside. You see in your mind a dark toxic trail escaping the car with the words "Parkinson's Disease" written upon it in white letters, diminishing into the sky. You shout, "Get out, Parkinson's! I have no room for you in my life! Go! Now!" Then you see it has all vanished to the air. (19)

Early in his slender book, Sel Kerans says that he wrote the book to share the good news: "We can do much to survive the onset of Parkinson's disease. It is possible to recover to a degree, to maintain health and independence; and delay or even reverse the effects of symptoms" (3). *Leading the Dance* is not for everyone, but isn't it nice to know that such optimists exist?

B24. *Shuffle: A Way Forward, Whatever the Challenge,* by Wendall Woodall. Charlotte, North Carolina: Highway 51 Publishing, 2014. v + 121 pp.

> "From the very beginning of my own struggle with Parkinson's, I've let the world know that I am going to face this with a large dose of honesty, and an even larger dose of humor."

Wendall Woodall, a teacher and assistant principal at a private school in North Carolina, was forty-nine when he began to notice that he was moving much more slowly and that his feet shuffled when he walked.

One day his daughter, home from college, watched him carry a glass and plate across the room. She asked him why he was walking like an old man. Her question sent him to his family doctor and then to a neurologist and finally to a movement disorder specialist who told him he had Parkinson's, a disease that was chronic, progressive, and incurable. That diagnosis inspired him to write *Shuffle* during the next three years.

Shuffle is different from most "my-journey-with-Parkinson's" books in that it says little about the medical or treatment aspects of the disease. Rather, it deals almost exclusively with the personal, psychological, emotional, and spiritual aspects. Instead of lamenting his diagnosis, Wendall Woodall saw his diagnosis as an opportunity to develop a meaningful plan for the rest of his life and to help others learn what he learned about what is most important in life:

> I want to share the emotions and thoughts that have filled my first 1000 days—the mere beginning of my path, I know—but also I hope to plot a course for my own heart and mind to follow from the very start. I welcome you along for the ride. I believe it was Confucius who said, "A journey of a thousand miles begins with a single shuffle." Well, at least that's what he would have said if he'd had Parkinson's, like me. (2)

Wendall Woodall's approach is very much that of a committed and practicing Christian. After college he worked as a pastor in a church in Florida, then he (with his wife and three daughters) spent a decade in Central America (mostly in Honduras) as a missionary, then taught and did administrative work at a private Christian school in Charlotte, North Carolina. He references both the Old Testament (especially Solomon) and the New Testament (especially Paul). For example:

> Like the Apostle Paul, we should do a little boasting about our weaknesses, maybe something like this: "I have Parkinson's, but that's not going to prevent me from doing what I feel like I'm supposed to do with my life. It may slow me down, perhaps considerably so, but I will not quit without even trying. Instead, I'm going to continue to fight against this condition every day of my life, the best I know how."
>
> I'm not talking about denial or some kind of motivational mumbo jumbo, nor am I advocating that we sugarcoat the reality of our unique conditions. In varying degrees, we all have physical and

mental limitations that we cannot simply ignore or pretend aren't there. No, I'm proposing that in the very face of those irrefutable and often limiting symptoms, we continue to shuffle forward, one day at a time, for as long as we possibly can. (24–25)

Wendall Woodall's message to his readers, however, is not all religion-oriented. He has a stimulating chapter of the six "habitudes" that he found helped him to cope most successfully with his Parkinson's: 1) dieting—to lose the extra twenty pounds he gained after his diagnosis; 2) exercising—to make up for the general slowness (bradykinesia) caused by his Parkinson's; 3) sleeping—to give him the energy to fight his disease symptoms when he was not sleeping; 4) reading—to keep himself informed and to keep his mind and spirit engaged; 5) volunteering—at a homeless kitchen to help others less fortunate than himself; and, 6) loving—particularly his wife and daughters, and letting them know how very much he appreciates all they do for him now and all they might need to do for him in the future.

For me the most engaging feature of *Shuffle* is the author's sense of humor. It is not merely that he makes little jokes about enjoying the game of shuffleboard. It is, rather, that humor is a central part of his whole approach to his Parkinson's:

From the very beginning of my own struggle with Parkinson's, I've let the world know that I am going to face this with a large dose of honesty and an even larger dose of humor. I believe the latter helps us swallow the former. So I laugh.

I laugh for my own sake and for the sake of my family and friends, to put them at ease from the start and to let them know they don't have to avoid any subjects around me. […] My wife and I wanted to come up with a nickname right away. She thought my "shuffling fool" moniker was too harsh, so we came up with "Shuffleupagus"—a tribute to a beloved character from our Sesame Street-watching days with our daughters and someone whose belabored movement and slow talk now seems warmly familiar. (No offense, Snuffleupagus.) The name stuck, as you can imagine, and every time we us it, it disarms people and they smile even if they don't think they should. […]

We explained that this was how we wanted to handle my condition—not with quiet whispers behind closed doors, but openly, freely, and … hilariously. It would be our way of saying that this thing hasn't beaten me and I intend to keep on living and enjoying life. (94–95)

Those paragraphs are from the next-to-last chapter, entitled "Humor." The last chapter is entitled "Hope." It ends with this sentence: "And hope keeps me shuffling forward, one tomorrow at a time, using every second wisely, trying not to waste a single day, focusing on the things that really matter" (121).

B25. *Tremors in the Universe: A Personal Journey of Discovery with Parkinson's Disease and Spirituality,* **by Robert Lyman Baittie. Bloomington, Indiana: Balboa Press, 2013. xv + 244 pp.**

> "Do the right thing, take a positive approach, and possess the faith that everything is going to work out well in the end. Keep in mind that happiness is a choice you can make regardless of your circumstances. Choose to be happy."

The first question that most readers of *Tremors in the Universe* will want to ask is what the title means. Robert Baittie explains it this way: it "just came to me. It felt right and it sounded right, and it couldn't have been more prophetic. Parkinson's has indeed shaken up my world. It's shaken me awake to the universe that is my life" (xiii). It is, of course, an awkwardly reductive leap to define "the universe" as "the universe that is my life," but that kind of leap is characteristic of Robert Baittie's approach to Parkinson's.

Tremors in the Universe began as a blog, sixteen months after graphic designer Robert Baittie got his Parkinson's diagnosis in 2012. Not surprisingly, *Tremors in the Universe* has the virtues and vices we might expect of a book that began as a blog. It has the refreshing immediacy of a here-is-what-I-am-thinking-about-today essay, but it also has the skip-around inconsistency of a journal. The individual chapters are often thoughtful and stimulating, but the overall trajectory of the argument is uncertain. Robert Baittie takes us from his diagnosis in his early fifties to his memories of a guardian angel who kept him from drowning when he was seven, to his not wanting his disease to cause him to be a burden to his family, to Michael J. Fox and his foundation, to his decision to volunteer for clinical trials, to his thought that the universe, if it were human, would be female, to a five-year-old girl who died of leukemia, to George Carlin, to the Beatles, to drugs used to treat the symptoms of Parkinson's, to his childhood rivalry with his older brother, to his decision to raise funds for Parkinson's research, to the time when, during a massage, his therapist saw the spirits of his grandfather and grandmother standing beside the massage table, to the Parkinson's "mask," to his three childhood concussions, to his problems with typing, to his trips with his kids, to his conviction that Parkinson's did not change him ("I am still the same person, with the same heart, the same smile and the same love of life" [123]), to—well, you get the idea.

Robert Baittie reports that he had three goals in writing this blog-book; 1) to give himself the chance to understand the relationship between his Parkinson's disease and his spirituality; 2) to help his three children understand their father's perspective on the disease; and 3) "to empower other Parkinson's patients with an honest, sincere, and inspirational view on living life positively with a chronic disease" (vii; rephrased on xiii). The first two of those goals are none of our business. It is only the third that I will address in this review. Do we other Parkinson's patients feel empowered by reading this book to live our lives with Parkinson's positively? My answer is, well, perhaps not.

Robert Baittie begins his life with Parkinson's with the intuitive conviction that "I can not only manage the disease but, with positive thoughts and attitudes that I draw from my spirituality, I can conquer it" (98). It is not clear in what sense he thinks he can "manage" and "conquer" Parkinson's. To be sure, he says, "I have every day physical reminders that tap me on the shoulder so that I will never forget that I have this disease. But rather than allowing those limitations to remind me of what Parkinson's is doing to me, I choose to remember I have the opportunity I've been given to fight against it—for myself and for others" (108). He is convinced that we can choose to be happy, even in hard times—"Anyone can make the choice to be happy" (213)—but he is somewhat vague about where his optimism comes from or what it means: "From the very first moment of my diagnosis, I have felt in my gut that I would be fine with my relationship with Parkinson's disease. Yet, in all honesty, I didn't know why or what that even meant. What does 'fine' mean?" (134).

Given that uncertainty, it is not clear what Robert Baittie's cheerful optimism—what his oft-asserted "positive attitude"—is based on. Apparently it is based partly on his conviction that all things happen for a reason: "It is my sincere belief that there is a reason behind everything that happens—negative experiences as well as positive" (135). Apparently this belief is based in part on his conviction that humans can choose to be happy or unhappy: "Where do I think my positive outlook comes from? There's really only one answer I've been able to come up with. It comes from choice—how I choose to look at life" (191). That is all well and good, but it is scarcely going to convince someone who does not already share that view. Many readers will wonder whether Robert Baittie has earned the right to generalize. It is easy enough for most people with Parkinson's disease to feel optimistic after having been diagnosed for only two-and-a-half years. Can they be blamed for wondering whether Robert Baittie will still feel so optimistic a decade later when his disease has progressed and when his meds are not so effective? "I've definitely found my peace with Parkinson's and I do trust everything will fall into place. And that gives me comfort" (135). We can hope, for his sake, that he will still feel so comfortable in 2025, a dozen years after his initial diagnosis.

Meanwhile, it seems premature, even cruel, for Robert Baittie to suggest that people who are unhappy with their Parkinson's are unhappy only because they *choose* to be unhappy. He closes his book with this advice to his readers: "Do the right thing, take a positive approach, and possess the faith that everything is going to work out well in the end. Keep in mind that happiness is a choice you can make regardless of your circumstances. Choose to be happy" (239). Is it really wise, is it really fair, to tell people who are feeling miserable with late-stage Parkinson's that they have *chosen* to feel miserable?

B26. *Everybody Has a Window and Aisle Seat: Choosing a Positive Approach to Parkinson's Disease*, by Mary Huston McLendon. Franklin, Tennessee: Cloverdale Publishing, 2015. 175 pp.

> "Get up, get unstuck, give back, and focus on living this wonderful life you have."

The first question a prospective reader will want answered about this book is what its title means. Mary Huston McLendon seems to believe that it is better to choose the window seat on the journey with Parkinson's:

> Every one of us has the choice between a window or aisle seat and choosing one or the other can make the trip frightening or

comforting. Taking the window seat keeps you focused outward
rather than inward, which lessens the possibility of feelings of
isolation, hopelessness, and despair. You can always get to the aisle
if need be. [...]

Sometimes when we focus so much on our ailments or issues,
we are tempted to get into the aisle seat, buckle up, and never
leave. [...] At times when we get so settled into the aisle seat we
get focused on our own little space. And we lose focus on the world
around us. Don't lose focus.

Get up, get unstuck, give back, and focus on living this
wonderful life you have. (13)

Mary McLendon explains her title with a story about an agent at the Delta
ticket counter in Baton Rouge who proudly announced that "everybody has
a window and aisle seat." The agent meant that it was a small airplane with
only one seat on either side of the aisle.

What are we to make of that story? Is the point that on that flight the
passenger really does NOT have a choice, in which case the advice to
choose the window seat is meaningless because the window and the aisle
seats are one and the same? Or is the point that people with Parkinson's are
best off being in a seat that permits us to look both inward and outward? Or
is the point that we should be in neither seat, but rather should "get up, get
unstuck," and leave the airplane? But if we are to do that, what does that do
to her advice, repeated at the end of the book: "Always choose a window
seat, and buckle up" (161). If everybody has both a window seat and an
aisle seat, what's to choose?

Everybody Has a Window and Aisle Seat is, like its title, unsure of its
direction. It is partly the author's memories of growing up in the South,
partly a Parkinson's log, partly advice to others with the disease, partly a
thank-you letter to her family, partly a poetic chapbook.

Mary McLendon had lived with a diagnosis of Parkinson's for almost
twenty years when she published her book. She tells us about it in long-line
couplets:

A Grim Diagnosis

The diagnosis was made with professionalism and much concern.
It is not every day that such devastating news a person will learn.

Parkinson's disease—I was way too young—I was just fifty-four.

I researched this disease (my disease) and learned much more.

Medications were available to slow down this progressive disease.
Without hesitation this was an option I was very quick to seize.

Living with Parkinson's gets harder each and every day.
And I listen to and do everything my doc has had to say (16–17).

There are more than 150 such lines in the book, some of them punctuated, most of them not. It is not clear why Mary McLendon tells some parts of her story in this prosaic verse, or what her notion of poetry is. Her idea of a couplet seems to be that two irregular lines of around a dozen to around twenty syllables constitute a stanza so long as they end in words that rhyme.

There is, however, much of interest in *Everybody Has a Window and Aisle Seat*. My own favorite parts are the deep brain stimulation (DBS) section (Chapters 15, 16, and 17) and the speech section (Chapter 19).

When her neurologist suggested that she consider the surgical option known as deep brain stimulation, Mary McLendon did a lot of research on what DBS would entail: drilling holes in her skull, inserting wires deep into her brain, embedding rechargeable batteries in her chest, then hooking them all up and flipping the on-switch. In the end, she says, the decision to try DBS was "really pretty simple. I had to do something and I had very little choice if I wanted a shot at delaying the most debilitating effects of Parkinson's" (108). She describes the evaluations, the anxiety, the drilling sounds "like a jack hammer" (113), the discomfort of "one awful headache" (113), the painful battery-implantation surgery which "felt like a huge truck had rolled over my chest" (117). Or, as she puts it in one of her poems:

My head is throbbing from electrodes in my brain bouncing to and
    fro.
And my chest muscles feel like I had a boob job with nothing to
    show. (117–18)

But all the discomfort was for Mary McLendon more than compensated for when they turned on the power in her DBS unit: "My tremors stopped almost immediately. [...] I literally skipped out of the medical center after arriving hobbling on a cane" (119). Would she make the decision to try DBS again? "You betcha. DBS gave me my life back." But she then adds the ominous warning: "For how long, nobody knows" (122).

My other favorite part of *Everybody Has a Window and Aisle Seat* is the chapter where Mary McLendon talks about the frustration of losing her ability to speak. We tend to think of Parkinson's as a movement disorder, a disease that slowly robs us of our ability to walk. Mary McLendon reminds us that even more frustrating for some of us is that it slowly robs us of our ability to talk. Let's hear about that frustration in her own voice:

> I was beginning to have issues when I talked. My voice had decreased in volume and I was difficult to hear, not what is ideal when your husband is very deaf and does not like to wear his hearing aids. Also, my hearing is so good, I feel like I am yelling while others say that is not the case. In addition to the softness of my voice, I was beginning to experience stuttering and also talking so fast that others could not understand what I said at times. (135)

She tried speech therapy, but did not have much success. She had some success slowing her speech down by tapping out the syllables when she talked, but she found that to be distracting to her listeners. She tried pausing every few words and taking a deep breath at the end of each sentence, but sometimes her auditors assumed that she was finished and would "steal the spotlight" by interjecting their own thoughts. She remained frustrated:

> In summary, speech therapy did not help much. This is the worst part of Parkinson's that I have had to face because I really don't have a feasible alternative for talking. My handwriting is illegible and I don't know sign language. A solution so far has been for me to use one word to get across my point when possible or prep my daughter or some other family member or friend so they can essentially translate for me. My good friends and members of my family will almost always try to help me by reading my lips, listening very intently, and generally letting me off the hook by finishing my sentences. This works OK but makes me feel like an incompetent stand-up comic. [...]
>
> Talking to people that I don't know well or to strangers really puts me in a twit. To speak or not to speak, that is the dilemma. My inclination is not to say much and when I do, I usually muddle through and leave them thinking that I am really "slow" or not all together, perhaps even a victim of a stroke or suffering from dementia. They may start to talk slowly so that I can understand and this gets me even more agitated and I talk faster because I want them

to understand what is going on. And boy, is it hard to try to explain all of this to someone unfamiliar with Parkinson's or the result of the disease. The bottom line is: What in the heck am I going to do? (136)

The answer to that question, for Mary Huston McLendon, was to write a book. This is that book.

B27. *If I Can Climb Mt. Kilimanjaro, Why Can't I Brush My Teeth?*: Courage, Tenacity, and Love Meet Parkinson's Disease, by Nan Little. Copyright 2015 by Nan Little. 232 pp.

> "We are in complete charge of our attitudes, but only to some limited extent, our disease."

Nan Little's name will be familiar to many as the driving force behind the Pedaling for Parkinson's program. She has been a frequent speaker at support groups and conferences. She has a doctorate in anthropology and is well-versed in Parkinson's. Her book is honest, brave, and not for the faint-hearted. If you want to read an optimistic, hope-saturated book about Parkinson's, *If I Can Climb Mt. Kilimanjaro*, may not be the book you want to reach for first.

"Parkinson's books tend to focus on positive aspects of having the disease," Nan Little tells us on the first page of her book:

> Whereas an upbeat attitude makes a huge difference in both slowing disease progression and determining how PwP's are "doing," a certain lie is embedded in this approach. Having an incurable disease, whether or not it's a neurodegenerative one like mine, is a bad deal. Prognosis, diagnosis, and reality tell us that over time the disease will worsen and the patient will become increasingly debilitated, quite possibly even demented. It's not a pretty prospect. No matter what resources a person has—intellectual, physical, financial, emotional, spiritual, or community-based—there is no denying that at some point the scales will tip in favor of the disease. (7)

The embedded "lie" that she finds at the heart of most of the cheerful and optimistic books about Parkinson's is that "if you just believe, and you try hard, you can do nearly anything. [...] I used to believe that was true" (7). And that is just the first page. It is almost a warning. Nan Little seems to be saying: if you want to feel uplifted, don't read my book.

But maybe you *should* read her book. It is the story of Nan Little's own amazing journeys, her unwillingness to sit still, her refusal to give up too early.

The answer to the question asked in the title *If I Can Climb Mt. Kilimanjaro, Why Can't I Brush My Teeth?* is of course Parkinson's. As with many book titles, the real subject of the book is revealed in the subtitle: *Courage, Tenacity, and Love Meet Parkinson's Disease.*

Courage. Anyone who has Parkinson's or is in a close relationship with someone who has it, knows about courage: the courage to get out of bed in the morning, the courage to get oneself dressed, the courage to appear in public, the courage to try to get some work done today. Nan Little writes about another kind of courage, the courage to ride a bike across the state of Iowa when she can scarcely walk to the start line, the courage to trudge to the frozen summit of the highest mountain in Africa, just to prove to herself and others that Parkinson's need not keep us from attempting to ascend to new heights.

Tenacity. Some people may find *If I Can Climb Mt. Kilimanjaro* to be a busy book, to be longer and more repetitive than it needs to be. Some will wonder why Nan Little comes back so often to the issue of biking, why she tells us not only about her life-altering first ride across Iowa in 2009, but also the rides she undertook in 2010, 2012, and 2014. They will understand why she tells us about her climb to the top of Mt. Kilimanjaro in 2011, but not why she also tells us about the details of her climb to Annapurna in 2012, and to Machu Picchu in 2013. One way to answer those concerns is to remind readers that dealing with Parkinson's demands tenacity. It was not just the first Iowa biking trip and the first mountain hiking trip that helped Nan Little manage her Parkinson's symptoms. It was the others as well. Dealing with Parkinson's is not doing something once and then knowing you're done. It is not like getting a knee replacement and then just getting on with your life. Parkinson's does not work that way. It persists. To fight its persistence requires tenacity. It means riding that bike again and again, climbing that mountain over and over.

Love. It is clear that love has been an important part of Nan Little's struggle with Parkinson's. Her husband Doug has struggled with her, supported her, encouraged her, teased her. And it is also clear that she is motivated in part to be as healthy as she can be so that she can be a help rather than a drag to the man she loves.

The most important features of *If I Can Climb Mt. Kilimanjaro* come at the end of the long section (chapters 14–16) on the Kilimanjaro climb. Does Nan Little think we should we all fly to Africa to climb Kilimanjaro? Of course not. We all already climb other Kilimanjaros every day:

> Every day of our lives—every day—we struggle to get up, to go swimming or dance or tai chi or whatever we do to get past our barriers. We struggle to ensure there is meaning in our lives. Every day, we PwP's climb a mountain higher than Mount Kilimanjaro—and no one is there to cheer. (141)

Nan Little speaks positively about the empowerment that comes from a fact-based attitude to our disease:

> People with Parkinson's can and should be empowered. We neither need to curl up and bemoan our diagnosis nor prove to anyone that we won't let our disease slow us down. Parkinson's will slow us down. Although perhaps we can be in control of our lives more than we are led to believe, the truth is that we have a progressive neurodegenerative disease that might be mitigated but won't be cured by medicine, exercise, or belief systems. We are in complete charge of our attitudes, but only to some limited extent, our disease. (138)

We can convince ourselves that the disease will go away by itself, the way a cold does, or that a cure is just around the corner. Or we can cheerfully accept the facts and be grateful that our disease moves slowly and gives us so many good years. And we should absolutely not feel guilty. It is not our fault that we got this disease. It is not our fault that our disease may adversely affect the people we love:

> When a person is told she can succeed if she only tries hard enough, there is an implicit underlying statement that if she does not succeed, she has not tried hard enough and somehow the failure rests in her, not in the course of the disease or something completely external. She is guilty if she fails. We have enough problems without adding guilt to the mixture. Stretching our goals is healthy. Beating ourselves up is not. (141)

The message of *If I Can Climb Mt. Kilimanjaro* is an important one: people with Parkinson's did nothing to deserve this disease. They can do a little, but only a little, to fight it. But they can change their attitudes. They can stop feeling guilty, stop feeling sorry for themselves, smile, and do what they can to make life more pleasant for those they love.

B28. *My Degeneration: A Journey Through Parkinson's*, by Peter Dunlap-Shohl. University Park: Pennsylvania State University Press, 2015. 96 pp.

> "What do you want from me?" […]
> "Everything. Everything it has taken you a lifetime to acquire, to learn, from buttoning your shirt to making music. […] Whatever you enjoy. […] I want it all, your entire self."

Peter Dunlap-Shohl was an editorial cartoonist, one of those journalists who draw witty caricatures of people in the news, usually making fun of them. He had fun doing that. Then, at age 43, the real fun began for Peter Dunlap-Shohl. He was diagnosed with early-onset Parkinson's disease. He discovered the fun of having trouble tying his shoes and buttoning his shirts, the fun of hearing his doctor say, "You have Parkinson's," the fun of words like "progressive," "disabling," and "incurable," the fun of finding out some of what lay ahead for him: loss of fine and gross motor skills, impaired ability to speak and swallow, loss of balance, and so on.

What did Peter Dunlap-Shohl do? He did what most of us do. He did what I call "futurize": he looked ahead and saw his life savings depleted by expensive doctors, nurses, and pharmaceutical bills, saw his family burdened by the care of a useless hunched, drooling, incontinent, wheelchair-trapped, twitching body. He flirted with suicide as a solution to the problem of a Parkinson's diagnosis. He decided to jog in a wooded area where bears had recently been sighted, hoping to be attacked and killed so that his wife and son would not know that he had taken his own life.

But then, like most of us, Peter Dunlap-Shohl came to his senses, listened to what his neurologist told him about diet, medicines, exercise, and support groups, listened to the soothing and sensible words of his spouse. He learned new meanings for old terms like "posture," "instability," "essential," "freezing," "frequency," "urgency," "accident," "falling," "tremor." He learned brand new vocabulary words like "agonist," "festination," "bradykinesia," "dyskinesia," "dystonia," "levodopa," "dopamine," "carbidopa." He learned that Parkinson's is a designer disease, different for each of us. He learned that certain things are good for all of us, like exercise, a Mediterranean diet, a positive attitude, and finding a congenial support group. And then he did what most of us do: he went to work to make a good life for himself and his family despite his diagnosis.

Peter Dunlap-Shohl exercised. He took his meds at the designated times. He continued to do things he liked to do, like camping. And he found a way to continue, at least for a time, his job at the newspaper. How does a witty editorial cartoonist whose hands shake so much that he cannot draw continue his job? He learned a computer program that let him continue to do his editorial cartooning. Fortunately for us, he decided to branch out from editorial cartooning and tell the story of his life with Parkinson's in a clever, colorful, and, yes, fun cartoon narrative. The result looks a little like a comic book, but it is longer and more serious than a comic book. It looks a little bit like a graphic novel, but it is not fiction and is mostly pictures, not prose. It is best described as an illustrated autobiographical essay the theme of which is, "I found a way to live with Parkinson's. You can too. And don't forget to be grateful."

The autobiographical essay, narrated mostly through cartoon pictures with captions, is compelling. The main character, Peter, appears in almost every cartoon frame. *My Degeneration* has eight chapters. The chapter titles suggest the author's growth in the course of his disease: 1. "Diagnosis Blues"; 2. "Learning to Speak Parkinson's"; 3. "Interview with a Killer"; 4. "Moping and Coping"; 5. "The Parkinson's Prism"; 6. "Island of the Caring and Competent"; 7. "A Different Path"; and 8. "Diagnosis, Reprise."

My own favorites are Chapters 3 and 6. In Chapter 3, "Interview with a Killer," Peter Dunlap-Shohl conducts an interview in his home with a sinister green-faced man named Parkinson's. Peter tells Parkinson's that lots of scientists are working hard "to nail you in a coffin." Parkinson's replies, "Hah! Good one! How many times have I heard people boast that I'll be gone in ten years?" (25). Peter then asks, "What do you want from me?" Parkinson's reply comes with a confident smirk: "Everything. Everything it has taken you a lifetime to acquire, to learn, from buttoning your shirt to making music, your ability to talk, to write legibly, even your ability to communicate non-verbally, to smile, to arch a brow. Whatever you enjoy, your work your income, your time, your marriage, your family. I want it all, your entire self, the physical and the emotional" (26). Then an angry-faced Parkinson's shakes his fist and says, "But here is all you need to know on the subject of me. I am Parkinson's disease! The thug who is going to kick your pathetic ass and leave it for the crows!" (28). Finally, Parkinson's leaves, but with these parting words: "Don't worry. I'll be back" (29). Grim stuff.

But things get better for Peter—and worse. He finds a way to keep working for a short time, until he goes out on disability. But enough good things happen that he is able to conclude that "I am one of the lucky of the unlucky" (59). He learns to appreciate what he calls "the finer miseries of Parkinson's" (60).

In Chapter 6, "Island of the Caring and the Competent," the once misanthropic and cynical cartoonist whose job it was to make people look evil and stupid is shipwrecked on an island peopled by good smart people who are out to help him. They help him get deep brain stimulation (DBS). They help him to understand that many, many good people are working hard to help him and others like him. He comes to appreciate

> the many researchers, caregivers, front-line neurologists, Parkinson's advocates, and family members. People who pour their skills, creativity, and passion into solving the endless riddles of Parkinson's disease. We can't yet celebrate a cure, but we sure should celebrate the people who bring the inevitability of that cure closer through their dedication, talent, and hard work. (83)

That sounds a bit cheerleaderish, especially in a book entitled *My Degeneration*, but Peter Dunlap-Shohl speaks for us all when he finds a way to say, "thank you."

B29. *Parkinson's Diva: A Woman's Guide to Parkinson's Disease,* **by Maria De León, MD. Copyright 2015 by Maria De León. xv + 286 pp.**

> "My mission would be complete if women with Parkinson's around the world become empowered, instead of paralyzed or panicked by the disease, through education, self-awareness, faith, and a desire to be a better advocate for themselves and others."

Who better than Dr. Maria De León could write a woman's guide to Parkinson's disease? She is a neurologist with years of experience in treating people—especially women—with Parkinson's. She helped to take care of her grandmother, who had Parkinson's. And she has Parkinson's disease herself. She was motivated to write this woman's guide to Parkinson's because she found that most books about Parkinson's talk about the disease in general terms, not recognizing that the disease can be quite different for women—especially younger women of childbearing age—whose chemistry is different. Their response to medicines is different. Their socio-economic situation is different. Their emotional and sexual needs are different. They are called on far more than men are to be caregivers, even though they themselves may also be in need of care. It is high time, Dr. De León says, for the medical world to stop treating women with Parkinson's—particularly young-onset women with Parkinson's—as if they were no different from old men with Parkinson's.

Clinical trials for medications, even for illnesses like migraines that are more common in women than in men, tend to enroll men, perhaps out of fear that a woman who later has a child with a birth defect may sue the drug company. Because there have been virtually no drug trials involving pregnant women with Parkinson's, neurologists simply do not know whether such mothers can safely be prescribed certain medicines. We have almost no evidence about the effect of the standard Parkinson's medications on nursing mothers or whether they have the same effect on pre- and post-menopausal women. Dr. De León thinks that "hormones are a big factor for why we see a wide variation in PD presentation, including age of onset, between men and women, but, more importantly, why women with PD seem to be more prone to develop 'negative' outcomes (such as job loss due to symptoms and a general discontent with quality of life) as well as an increase in non-motor symptoms, such as depression" (27).

Dr. De León is refreshingly honest about sensitive issues such as sexuality. In Chapter 9, "Sex and Parkinson's: The Bedroom Goddess," she says this:

> Sexual issues can be a huge problem in any marriage or partnership, but even more critical in people living with PD when nearly eighty-seven per cent of people with this disorder professed to having some type of sexual problem according to a survey of 351 PD patients. Furthermore, because of its personal nature it is something that has to be dealt with, not just in a timely manner but also very delicately, to avoid issues of guilt, self-doubt, blame, loss of self-esteem, or even self-deprecation in either partner. (83–84)

Dr. De León specifically mentions the Parkinson medicine called Azilect, which can contribute to vaginal and bladder problems: "Hence it can be extremely hard to be the sex diva your mate wishes or that you envision when you have constant bladder issues, vaginal irritation, or irregular menses due to Parkinson's" (105). She defines the word "diva" as "a lady of distinction and good taste" and explains that the word derives from the Latin and Italian words for "goddess, fine lady" (iv). Her use of the term "diva" in her title may be partly jocular, but not entirely.

She gives practical advice on all sorts of issues of interest to women with Parkinson's: how to put on makeup when your hands shake, what kind of shoes to buy so you don't have to tie them, how to fasten your bra when you cannot reach back there anymore.

A woman who has Parkinson's and who wants to have a child has much to consider: is Parkinson's hereditary?; are there special risks for her unborn child?; can she take her meds while she is pregnant?; will she likely have a normal delivery?; will being pregnant make her Parkinson's worse?; should she breast-feed the baby, and if she does, can she continue to take her Parkinson's medications?; will she live long enough to see her child become an adult?; can she or should she have a second child?; when and how should she tell her child that she has Parkinson's?; will having children put exceptional strains on her marriage?

Women with Parkinson's have unique problems when the going gets rough. Often they are saddled with financial burdens greater than those that men face. They are paid less than men, have more responsibility caring for their parents than their brothers have, more responsibility for caring for their children than their [ex]husbands have, and they live longer and so have greater medical expenses. If their husbands get a chronic illness, women are usually willing to take care of them. On the other hand, "when a woman, especially a young woman, suddenly takes ill with a chronic, progressive, debilitating, neurodegenerative disease, for which there is no cure, most men simply state they are ill-equipped to handle this life-challenge, some reiterating 'they did not sign up for this,' and so they simply bow out" (2–3).

Dr. De León wrote *Parkinson's Diva* because she hoped to inspire better treatment for women who have Parkinson's. She hoped to guide "other women on this journey, to help them become empowered with fellowship and knowledge, and to encourage female participation in the research that will ultimately affect our overall quality of life and wellbeing" (xi). "My mission would be complete," she goes on, "if women with Parkinson's around the world become empowered, instead of paralyzed or panicked by the disease, through education, self-awareness, faith, and a desire to be a better advocate for themselves and others" (xiii).

Dr. De León is, after all, a hopeful person: "I still believe in the promise of a better tomorrow for those who suffer many neurological illnesses like Parkinson's. The hope is to one day find a cure for Parkinson's. With your help and participation and with our growing scientific knowledge, which can be molded and inspired by you, we CAN find a CURE!" (12).

B30. *Tenacity: A Memoir*, by Jonathan Lessin, MD. Hidden Thoughts Press, 2015. xi + 103 pp.

> "Merely being around others with PD can make some of our symptoms improve tremendously. Some people may begin to speak more clearly. […] I skied the best I ever had since my diagnosis."

The director of anesthesiology residency at MedStar Washington Hospital Center, Dr. Jonathan Lessin, who was also an assistant professor of anesthesiology at Georgetown University Medical School, was just thirty-eight when he was diagnosed with young-onset Parkinson's disease. He had known for some time that something was wrong: he was clumsy, his coordination was off, he had tremors in his hands, he slouched, he walked leaning forward, slowly and stiffly. One doctor thought he had multiple sclerosis, but that diagnosis did not pan out.

Dr. Lessin's reaction when he was finally told it was Parkinson's disease was relief: "I actually smiled. Now we had a disorder, and we could treat it" (28). Instead of wondering what in the world was wrong, he now had a name for what was wrong. He could read about it and ask about it. He found out that Parkinson's was usually not hereditary, that certain medicines were effective in treating its symptoms, that he could continue to work, and that the disease would probably not shorten his life.

Dr. Lessin continued to work as a cardiac anesthesiologist for several years after his diagnosis, but then he began to have further difficulties. He discovered a wearing-off of his medicines when he ingested protein-rich foods, and he started to have freezing of gait. He turned in his resignation letter and went on disability. He learned about a brain surgery known as deep brain stimulation and decided to have it done. His DBS surgery was amazingly successful. When the surgeon flipped the switch sending electrical pulses into is brain, Dr. Lessin suddenly felt wonderful: "He turned it on, and I felt amazing. My whole brain was awake! I felt light as a feather. I jumped up, stretched my arms above my head, and began to run around the clinic" (41).

Readers who are mostly interested in finding out more about Parkinson's will particularly want to read Chapters 6 through 9 (about ten percent of the book). The rest of the text wanders around a bit: Dr. Lessin's family's emigration from Europe, his own experiences with schoolyard bullies, his wilderness trek as a teenager in Canada, his courtship of Cheryl, their two daughters, his decision to be a doctor and to specialize in anesthetics.

Then after the DBS chapter, his story wanders around in different directions: his decision to retire from his job and take disability, his decision to learn how to fly an airplane, his taking up bicycling, his hiking with his daughter along a dangerous trail above a Potomac River gorge, his taking up skiing and hot-room yoga, his enrolling in an LSVT BIG training program, and his starting a rock-climbing club for people with Parkinson's.

Some of these ventures relate pretty well to Parkinson's. In chapter 15, for example, entitled "A House Full of Parkies," Dr. Lessin described his decision to join a dozen other "Parkies"—his perhaps-too-flippant word for people with Parkinson's—at an outdoor education center in Breckenridge, Colorado. The idea was to make it possible for people with Parkinson's, even the ones who were wheelchair-bound, to ski. What was most interesting to me in that chapter was not how non-ambulatory patients could be fitted with special harnesses or other equipment that allowed them to experience the thrill of skiing, but what Dr. Lessin learned while sharing a cabin with a dozen other men and women with the disease:

> There was something about living together that was liberating. We Parkies understood each other's struggles and issues beyond our control, such as snoring or screaming while asleep, for example. There also exists a phenomenon whereby merely being around others with PD can make some of our symptoms improve tremendously. Some people may begin to speak more clearly. I skied the best I ever had since my diagnosis. Some people conjecture that this occurs because we are not self-conscious, so there is less cortical input and more old ingrained memory guiding our actions. [...] We are all in this together. Every Parkie in the world is on the same team. Sometimes it just takes someone who understands what you are going through to make you feel better. (66, 68)

One of the most puzzling features of *Tenacity* is the way Dr. Lessin has framed his memoir into four sections, each introduced by a portion of the "perseverance" narrative of his five-week adventure as a sixteen-year-old boy on a wilderness canoe journey, with four others, in the wilds of northern Canada. I suppose the idea is that that life-altering experience with perseverance helped to prepare him for dealing with Parkinson's later on. It also helps to explain his lifelong need to risk his life by doing things that not many people with Parkinson's can safely do: hiking, leaping, flying, rock climbing, and so on. The fourth section of his wilderness perseverance narrative—the section about his finding a moose carcass in the woods and the attempt to bring it back as a trophy of some sort seems especially opaque. We understand that the canoe carrying the antlered skull capsized and forced him and his companions to leave it at the bottom of a river in Canada, but it is not clear to me what that has to do with Parkinson's.

It is difficult for any writer to know how or when to bring to an end the story he or she is telling. Dr. Lessin seems to have a particularly difficult time with that. The story trails off into his reprinting self-serving letters that his resident trainees wrote to him on the occasion of his retirement. They say over and over what a good mentor he was to them. Put together with other bits about the many lives he saved as a doctor, his closing of his book with those letters seems to suggest a need to assure himself by assuring others that his life had mattered. If so, it may suggest the toll that Parkinson's disease takes from many of us by making us wonder whether our disease has kept us from being all that we might have been had the disease not slowed us down.

Dr. Lessin might better have ended his book with Chapter 22, "What's Really Important":

> Dealing with Parkinson's disease has taught me to appreciate what's really important in life. We share this Earth with over seven billion people, and I think we all find positive human interaction to be the most important thing. It's so easy to get caught up in the consumer phase of life, competing for the most respected profession, and the best schools for your kids, the big house, and a nice car. Everybody is trying to get their piece of the pie—and make it a big one. We are taught by society that this is the key to happiness. None of these things, however, correlates with real fulfillment. Helping people smile or get relief from seemingly insurmountable struggles is why we are actually here. The happiest people are those with the most love in their lives. Luckily Parkinson's disease is not contagious, but a smile is. (91)

Having Parkinson's does make us reassess what is really important. We all have different ideas about what that is: writing a novel, serving others, asking forgiveness, falling in love, traveling, going back to school, whatever. Go for it, and go with tenacity.

B31. *The Day I Found Out Why: My Life's Journey with Parkinson's Disease*, by Israel Robledo. Copyright 2016 by Israel Robledo. 207 pp.

"The worries of living and dealing with an incurable disease seemed to disappear because it was then that I made a promise to myself to do what I could, while I still could, to make a difference."

The forty-two-year-old Israel Robledo, a special education teacher in Midland, Texas, was already troubled by the darkness of depression when he was diagnosed with Parkinson's in 2007. That diagnosis, and the voracious reading that he did after receiving it to find out about the disease, "turned out to be the start of the darkest period of my life" (51). Although his book, which draws on a journal he kept, a blog he started, and his life as an advocate for various causes relating to Parkinson's disease, is deeply personal; it is meant to help others deal with the darkness of Parkinson's by showing them how he dealt with it.

Israel Robledo sees his book as falling into two parts. In the first part he sets out to show that a diagnosis of Parkinson's "is not the end of the world (although it sure does feel like it at first)" (19). He quotes from his journal:

> I've set out to write my thoughts, emotions, and otherwise sad details of this life sentence. A life sentence without the possibility of parole. How does a seemingly healthy individual one day become a person with an incurable disease? [...] The underlying turmoil is what takes over when the internal tremors are uncontrollable and the balance is off and you're afraid to move so as not to risk falling. (20–21)

The solution to this turmoil, he says, is to keep alive your hope for a cure:

> To lose hope is to stop living. I've always said that if I stop dreaming I stop living. My dream is of a cure like that for Polio. A grand entrance to the final dance knowing that we've done our part to make this disease a thing of the past. A way of life no longer to be. No more suffering and being able to feel 'normal' again. Oh, what a joyful day that will be! (22–23)

In the second part of his book the author describes his own efforts to keep that dream alive by engaging in what he calls advocacy. That takes us to the meaning of the title of the book. It turns out that the title comes from a statement by Mark Twain: "The two most important days in your life are the day you were born, and the day you found out why" (quoted on p. 7). For Israel Robledo, that all-important second day was the day that he decided that he was born to become an advocate for people with Parkinson's by fighting for a cure, by raising consciousness about the disease, and by helping to raise money for research. Finding out why he was born made all the difference to him:

> The worries of living and dealing with an incurable disease seemed to disappear because it was then that I made a promise to myself to do what I could, while I still could, to make a difference. It was no longer just about me dealing with this disease. There were many more people who were worse than me whom [sic*] had no support of any kind. That moment, on that day, became the starting point of an incredibly fulfilling journey of a lifetime. (94–95)

[* As a retired English professor, I could not help noticing the couple of dozen places where, like here, the author misuses "whom." For example, he dedicates his book "To some special people whom have been placed in my work life and have, each in their own way, been a blessing to me on this journey" (10).]

Much of the second part of the book is inspirational, but at times it starts to sound dangerously close to bragging about all of the committees Israel Robledo served on, all of the conferences he attended, and all of the people he befriended.

This book has useful information about the various organizations for treating and researching Parkinson's disease: Parkinson's Disease Foundation (PDF), World Parkinson's Coalition (WPC), Parkinson's Movement (PM), Parkinson's Action Network (PAN), Patient-Centered Outcomes Research Institute (PCORI), Michael J. Fox Foundation, Davis Phinney Foundation, and so on. Israel Robledo has been especially interested in raising funds, through his own non-profit called Parkinson's Outreach, for people who cannot afford to see a doctor or pay for medications. He has also worked hard to persuade people doing and funding clinical trials to provide funds to cover the transportation costs of patients who do not live near the physical site of the research. He openly and enthusiastically encourages others, whether they have Parkinson's themselves or not, to become active advocates by telling their stories, contributing funds, helping advance research, and working for a cure.

Israel Robledo demonstrates a winning, if sometimes naive, enthusiasm for his dream of a cure, but he also seems to suspect that some researchers may be secretly ambivalent about actually finding a cure because they will then be out of work: "I have made a promise on several occasions that I will spend the rest of my life, after being cured of PD, seeking meaningful employment for these people who find the cure" (177–78). Near the end of *The Day I Found Out Why*, he admits to a certain disappointment at not having achieved more: "I look back on some of the things that I've done to help out and I find myself not being too happy with the outcome. Until we find new treatments that impact the majority of the PD community or we find a cure, whatever that may mean for all of us, I don't think I'll be satisfied with my work as an advocate" (183).

I close with this message to Israel Robledo: The cure you have set your sights on is elusive indeed. It may come too late to help you personally, or it may come in a form that may sound more like "a way to avoid getting Parkinson's in the first place" than "a way to cure Parkinson's once you have it," but know this: that it came about through the advocacy of a couple of generations of indefatigable and devoted people like you. Thank you, Israel.

B32. *Faces of Parkinson's: Global Reflections on PD.* Copyright 2016 by The World Parkinson Coalition. 69 pp.

> "Parkinson's is a reminder that every moment is precious, and to be used wisely while keeping hope alive."

In the third week of September 2016, over 4500 people from 67 countries gathered in Portland, Oregon, to attend the fourth World Parkinson's Congress. Those who registered early received this website post:

> The World Parkinson's Congress is looking for registrants to apply to participate in a special project at the WPC 2016 in September. To be considered for the project, please submit in 200 words or less, the impact Parkinson's has had on your life or how your life changed

because of your association to Parkinson's, whether as a researcher, clinician, or person living with it.

The review committee received 147 submissions. Of these, the editorial committee selected sixty-three—fewer than half of those submitted—to be published in a short book. The committee arranged for the people whose statements they had selected to have their photographs taken at the World Parkinson's Congress in Portland. The completed book, *Faces of Parkinson's*, came out just before Christmas, 2016.

Among those whose statements were printed under their photographs, nearly two-thirds (thirty-nine) were written by people with the disease. Most of the rest were written by clinicians, researchers, and advocates (sixteen), by partners and family members (four), by artists (four) who use art, music, and dance to help people with Parkinson's. I select for brief quotation here only from the large group of thirty-nine people with Parkinson's. Most of those, while admitting to the limitations and frustrations that the disease brought into their lives, have far more to say about how they have benefitted from their disease. I provide exemplary bits from only a few of the thirty-nine:

—"I went from 'Why me?' to 'I'm blessed' in an incredible on-going journey that has re-oriented me from a materialistic perspective to a spiritual mindset. It has made me more empathetic, sympathetic, and calmer" (7).

—"Rather than lament the loss, I find myself counting my blessings. I meet amazing people with Parkinson's. I have deepened my understanding of patience and compassion for others" (8).

—"Despite Parkinson's hassles and horrors, I am thankful because the disease forces me to live life fully" (10).

—"Parkinson's is a reminder that every moment is precious, and to be used wisely while keeping hope alive" (13).

—"Parkinson's disease is a gift. [...] Without PD [...] I wouldn't have experienced the miracle of deep brain stimulation. [...] Simply put, my life suddenly began to hold more meaning" (15).

—"This has made me more compassionate, less intolerant of others' difficulties" (18).

—"The first feeling I had when I was diagnosed with PD at the age of sixty was relief. I had an excuse to not ever return to work" (20).

—"This PD twist in my journey was unexpected; however, I am thankful for the people I have had the privilege to encounter and for the opportunity to join with them to make a difference" (33).

—"It has made me aware of my mortality and the need to leave happy memories to my children, grandchildren, and my great grandson" (38).

—"It has allowed me not to take things for granted and live life to the fullest" (42).

—"A slight tremor appeared in my hand. I was nervous and a little scared; three months later I was diagnosed with Parkinson's disease. I was a little shocked that Tony and I both felt relieved. I didn't know where the road would take me, but it did have a name. I am happy to say that the road is now a bright new path" (44).

—"I bought myself a motorcycle, as the idea of living out dreams seemed to come with a time-clause. PD has made me live more intensely, more real, and more Now" (48).

—"I am suddenly no longer the smart, relevant person I once was. Often clerks and receptionists will talk to my husband instead. 'Does she need anything?' I went from larger than life to invisible" (12).

—"PD changed me into a more patient and more compassionate person. I wouldn't go back" (66).

—"If you're looking for words or stories of inspiration, you won't find them here. I'm tired of being inspired" (17).

—"I am the eighth (possibly ninth) member [of my family] to suffer from this horrible disease" (28).

—"I treat Parkinson's with the contempt it deserves" (47).

—"PD ruins my dreams for the future. PD teaches me to live in the present. […] PD shows me that helping others helps myself.

[…] PD makes me think, how am I going to avoid burdening others? What money will be left for my kids? […] PD is a curse and a gift" (51).

—"I came to the realization that life with Parkinson's was just a new beginning, not the beginning of the end" (60).

—"If I think only about the future, I'll curl up and cry. I plan for the future, but I only think now. […] I'm not going to beat PD—I'm a realist. But I can choose not to let it destroy me—not yet" (65).

If these people with Parkinson's were not thoughtful people they would not have gone to the trouble and expense of attending the World Parkinson's Congress in Portland. If they were not serious about their disease, they would not have submitted statements for inclusion in *Faces of Parkinson's*. Because they did both, their serious thoughts about dealing with Parkinson's are well worth reading.

B33. *Old Age: A Beginner's Guide*, by Michael Kinsley. New York: Tim Duggan Books, 2016. 157 pp.

"If you're going to get a serious disease—and unless you'd prefer to die violently and young, you're probably going to—Parkinson's is not your worst choice."

Why am I writing for people interested in Parkinson's disease about a book by an author who announces in his opening sentence that "This is not a book about Parkinson's disease"? The answer is that in *Old Age* Michael Kinsley really does have a lot to say about Parkinson's, a disease he has lived with for the past quarter-century. There is other stuff in *Old Age*—about the baby boomer generation of Americans born between 1946 and 1964, about why and how they should pay down the national debt, and about how to ensure that you will be remembered after you are dead—but even those parts are informed by the experience of a man who knows that he will die with, if not of, Parkinson's.

Michael Kinsley is a well-known journalist who writes with authority, statistical integrity, and humor about what he knows. One of the things he knows about is Parkinson's. In what follows, the questions are mine; the answers are Kinsley's.

How bad is it to have Parkinson's?

Answer: "If you're going to get a serious disease—and unless you'd prefer to die violently and young, you're probably going to— Parkinson's is not your worst choice. [...] Like its victims, it tends to move slowly. It is not generally considered fatal—meaning that there's enough time for something else to get you first" (19). "There are far worse medical conditions than Parkinson's" (68). "[My] bad back has been more burdensome to me than Parkinson's" (87).

Cancer and heart disease are the number one and two killer diseases in the United States. What number is Parkinson's disease?

Answer: Number fourteen. "Not only do most people with Parkinson's not die of it, but even of those who do, almost half make it past eighty-five." (62). "My chance of being alive at eighty [...] is about as good as that of any other sixty-five-year-old American male. That chance is almost exactly fifty-fifty. And I'm more likely to be felled by a heart attack [...] than by Parkinson's" (67–68).

Is it accurate to describe Parkinson's as a "movement disorder"?

Answer: "How could experts have failed to notice until the past two decades that Parkinson's is as much about cognitive problems as it is about physical ones? In fact, I would say that there are three categories of Parkinson's symptoms: physical symptoms, such as shaking or freezing; cognitive symptoms, such as the number of states you can name in thirty seconds (go!), and psychiatric symptoms, such as depression" (94).

How prevalent are the cognitive and psychiatric symptoms associated with Parkinson's?

Answer: Kinsley cites Patrick McNamara, a neurologist at Boston University: "Upwards of 85% of PD patients evidence deficits in executive cognitive functions even early in the disease. [...] More than half of all patients suffer severe anxiety or depression" (91).

Is Kinsley glad that he had the brain surgery called deep brain stimulation (DBS)?

Answer: "This surgery has been a miracle in terms of reducing the physical symptoms of Parkinson's" (104).

Is it sensible for us to want to live as long as possible?

Answer: "Anyone who lives past eighty-five, as more and more of us intend to, has roughly a fifty-fifty chance of exiting by way of Alzheimer's. So there are two forms of competition in the boomer death-style Olympics. There's dying last and there's dying lucid. [...] If you're prepared to die at sixty, you can pretty much scratch dementia off your list of things to worry about. By contrast, if you don't mind being a bit dotty—or worse than that—you can go for longevity. But unless you're extremely lucky, you won't win at both games" (85–86).

So what is so bad about dementia?

Answer: "There is a special horror about the prospect of shuffling down the perennially unfamiliar corridors of some institution in a demented fog, being treated like a child by your children, watching TV all day but unable to follow even the most simpleminded propaganda on Fox News or the most facile plot twist of *Downton Abbey*. Dementia seems like an especially humiliating last stop on the road of life" (83).

Should our goal be to live the most years or to live with the most marbles?

Answer: "So 'Death before dementia' is your rallying cry. It is also your best strategy, at the moment, since there's no cure for either one" (85).

How does the dementia associated with Alzheimer's differ from the dementia associated with Parkinson's?

Answer: "Alzheimer's tends to start its destruction in the parts of the brain affecting memory, whereas Parkinson's starts with what they call the executive function: analyzing a situation and your options and making a decision" (97).

Should people with Parkinson's be concerned about falling?

Answer: "Pneumonia used to be called 'the old man's friend' because it ended so many lives whose owners were finished with them. That role (though possibly not the label) has now been taken over by accidental falls. The death rate from falls nearly doubled from 30 per 100,000 in the year 2000 to nearly 60 per 100,000 in 2013" (60).

See, *Old Age* really is about Parkinson's.

B34. *Power over Parkinson's: How to Live Your Best Life Even after Your Parkinson's Disease Diagnosis*, by Terry Cason. San Bernardino, California, 2016. 304 pp.

> "Just because you have this disease doesn't mean you should give up, crawl in the corner, and let life pass you by."

Terry Cason is a freelance writer who at the end of 2012, at age forty-eight, was diagnosed with Parkinson's disease. He was not at all happy about it. He shopped around to different doctors hoping to find a friendlier diagnosis, but eventually had to accept the fact that he had Parkinson's. Why did he get it? He is not sure, but "I have to believe that there's a reason behind it. […] I believe that I developed this horrible disease so I could use my experience to help others who have also been diagnosed" (12). *Power over Parkinson's*, the tangible result of that belief, is available in paperback from Amazon.com, but it has no title page, lists no publisher, and gives no page numbers. I hand-numbered the pages in my copy so that I could reference my quotations.

Keeping in mind that his purpose is to help people recently diagnosed with Parkinson's, Cason organizes much of what he says around a dozen "insights" that he wishes he had known about when he was newly diagnosed. I list them here along with brief quotations.

> **Insight # 1**: Your life isn't over (13). "Just because you have this disease doesn't mean you should give up, crawl in the corner, and let life pass you by. There's absolutely no reason why you shouldn't plan on living just the same as you would if you didn't have Parkinson's" (14).

> **Insight # 2**: Share your diagnosis with others (18). "The more people you open up to, the better you'll be able to handle it yourself" (18).

Insight # 3: Everybody progresses at different rates (57). "Most patients may have already advanced to the second or sometimes even the third stage of Parkinson's by the time they reach a diagnosis. This doesn't mean you're too late to do anything about it so don't ever let your mind go there. It does mean that you need to be proactive about your treatment because the clock is ticking … ticking … ticking … With Parkinson's disease, it's always ticking" (58).

Insight # 4: Protein affects your medications (81). "Parkinson's patients have a unique situation when it comes to eating protein because having too much of it or having it at the wrong times can interfere with their medications. […] Instead of crossing protein out of your meals completely, a better option for consuming protein is to take it at least thirty minutes before or at least one and preferably two hours after a meal. But the best option, by far, is to limit your intake of protein throughout the day as much as possible so you don't have to worry about keeping up with the timing" (81, 83).

Insight # 5: Caffeine can make your symptoms worse (93). "While there are some scientists who theorize that caffeine can actually help to reduce the risk of developing Parkinson's disease, that doesn't really offer much help to those of us who have already been diagnosed" (93).

Insight # 6: Keep your cholesterol levels up (96). "Scientists […] discovered irrefutable proof that there was an obvious connection between low cholesterol and the occurrence of Parkinson's disease. You read that right: low cholesterol" (96).

Insight # 7: Eat balanced meals (102). "Proper nutrition is one of the best things you can do to help manage your disease" (102).

Insight # 8: Get tested for food and especially gluten sensitivity (103). "As I weaned off of gluten, I began to realize that gluten had been amplifying my symptoms. Even worse, it was accelerating the progression of the disease due to the fact that it was attacking my brain" (115).

Insight # 9: It is really hard to get good sleep (150). "No one knows how difficult it is to get good sleep more than someone with

Parkinson's (a close second would be the person who has to sleep in the same bed with someone who has Parkinson's)" (150).

Insight # 10: Genetic testing can be beneficial (189). "Research has shown us that roughly one in every ten cases of Parkinson's can be linked back to genetics" (189).

Insight # 11: There may be ways to slow the progression of Parkinson's (215). "There are many alternative treatment options available for Parkinson's patients that have the potential of helping reduce the effects of the disease and give you a better quality of life. Notice I said 'potential.' There are no guarantees" (215).

Insight # 12: Exercise is important (287). "You already know that Parkinson's is a degenerative disease so it only gets worse as time goes on. You also know that eating right, taking the proper supplements, getting good, quality sleep and keeping stress down to a minimum all play a major part in the big picture of slowing down the progression of the disease and helping to keep symptoms under control. You've likely also heard that exercise is important, too, for helping fight off the attacks from Parkinson's. Well, as important as those other points are, that last one may just well be the understatement of the century" (253).

Power over Parkinson's is generally well-written and clear, and the advice it offers to the newly diagnosed is generally sound. My main hesitation in recommending it is its author's belligerent stance. At the start of his book Cason urges patients to think of themselves as warriors fighting an enemy: "if you decide to take a stand and fight back with everything you can do to slow the progression, then you'll live a longer, happier, and more productive life. [...] If you fight back, kicking and screaming, you have the ability to make a huge difference. It's all up to you" (19). Near the end of his book Cason asserts that exercise is important because it helps patients "fight off the attacks from Parkinson's" (253). Cason's closing line in the book is, "Stay strong and I wish you all the best in your fight against Parkinson's disease!" (302). But is it really helpful to newly-diagnosed patients to insist that they see Parkinson's as an evil, powerful enemy who needs to be fought? Might it not be better to suggest a different metaphor than the military one? For example, might we encourage newly-diagnosed patients to think of themselves less as warriors than as teachers who are trying to understand the schoolyard bully, that big kid over there who is trying to intimidate the little kids? Alternatively, might we encourage the newly diagnosed to think of themselves as biomedical researchers trying to understand a dangerous virus?

B35. *Shake, Rattle, and Roll with It: Living and Laughing with Parkinson's* (second edition), by Vikki Claflin. Mill Creek Publishing, 2016. xi + 215 pp.

> "If I was going to live with this for the next twenty-thirty years, I was decidedly not going to spend it trudging through the five stages of grief. [...] For me, laughter was the only suitable response to what was coming."

Vikki Claflin, who lives in Hood River, Oregon, is a delight. A professional humorist and blogger, she has spent much of her adult life writing funny things about her life and times. When she was diagnosed with Parkinson's a half-dozen years ago, like most of us she tried to keep it a secret for a while. And she succeeded. For a while. Then one day a friend said to her, "So when will you write about your Parkinson's?" Vikki whispered, "You knew?" "Well, yes. [...] Vikki, your Parkinson's is part of your story. An important part. It's real. And it's the truth. How would it be if you wrote about it?" (xiii). The following Monday Vikki Claflin came out in her blog about her Parkinson's. Since then, she has been writing funny things about a not very funny disease.

Vikki Claflin readily admits that she exploits her personal experiences to make people laugh: "I have somewhere near zero reservations about offering my personal humiliations for public amusement" (78). How funny is it when she makes a mess trying to eat noodles with a shaky hand? Well, it is *this* funny:

> Grabbed a fork and spent the next two minutes trying to guide my noncompliant tremor hand into the general direction of my plate, until I finally managed to stab a macaroni elbow, hopefully securing it on the fork tines long enough to get it to my mouth. [...] Four tries later, with two macaroni noodles in my hair and half a dozen tremor-launched onto the floor or down the front of my shirt, it appeared I

was going to starve to death, until surprisingly, I hit my target. Sort of. I had two noodles in my mouth. I also stabbed myself in the lip and on my cheek, bleeding all over my fork. (78–79)

Vikki Claflin's humor will probably appeal especially to women readers. Here she is describing what it is like trying to wiggle her middle-aged hips into a Spanx girdle:

My undergarments had become less frivolous and more functional. Less about wisps of lace whispering "Hey, Sailor, new in town?" and more about lifting, stuffing, and otherwise coaxing recalcitrant areas into clothes I used to wear with ease. And Parkinson's brings its own list of challenges to the Spanx table. Simply put, if you struggled with Spanx before you got Parkinson's, you now need to add an extra twenty minutes to your morning routine. Reduced grip strength and balance issues can make these almost insurmountable. […] I spent the next fifteen minutes wriggling, cramming, and yanking the tightly knit miracle worker into place. First, you yank it up on one side, alternating with a "hop-wiggle" to shimmy it into position, then repeat on the other side, alternating until you're saddled up and ready to ride. (91)

She goes on to describe the funny time she toppled over with the Spanx halfway on and had to let her husband help her get back on her feet. She concludes by asserting that "Spanx, while unparalleled in terms of cramming a size 10 butt into size 8 pants, were not designed for Parkinson's patients" (102). Especially not women, like her, who were klutzes to start with: She admits, almost with pride, that she was an awkward, stumbling klutz, even before Parkinson's: "Give a klutz Parkinson's, and she'll spend more time on the floor than standing up" (114). What makes all this funny is that she thinks it's funny. If others wrote such things about her we would all think they were being cruel. They become funny only because she has found a way to let us know that she thinks they are funny. It is hard to write a funny book about an unfunny disease. Only someone with Parkinson's could pull it off, but even as we laugh with her, our laughter may feel a bit forced.

My own favorite chapters are ones I would describe as witty rather than funny. There is wit enough in Vikki Claflin's chapter on "Thirteen Things NOT to Say to a Parkinson's Patient." She admits that it is difficult to know what to say to someone with Parkinson's, but she speaks from experience when she says that some things are "virtually guaranteed to offend" (174). For example:

> 1. "Why are you shaking?" Unless you are five years old, this is just plain rude. [...]
>
> 2. "Do you have Parkinson's?" If you don't know, we're not close enough for you to be asking that question. [...]
>
> 3. "Can you make it stop?" Assuming that you're referring to the tremors, uh ... no. If I could, I would. [...]
>
> 4. "There's no cure, right?" No, and thank you for reminding me. [...]
>
> 7. "My grandfather had Parkinson's, and was in a wheelchair until he died last year." [...]
>
> 10. "You should quit drinking Diet Coke. That's probably why you got Parkinson's." [...]
>
> 12. "God never gives us more than we can handle." [...]
>
> 13. "Everything happens for a reason." [...] (175–77)

There is a good chapter entitled "Hubs Speaks Out"—a loving expression of gratitude for the good things her husband has said and done about the disease she has but that they share (see 181–85).

Mostly, though, *Shake, Rattle, and Roll with It* is about the wisdom of laughter as a response to Parkinson's:

> If I was going to live with this for the next twenty-thirty years, I was decidedly not going to spend it trudging through the five stages of grief. Denial was over. Anger was a waste. Bargaining seemed fruitless (I already had the disease). Depression was so ... well, sad. Acceptance was an option if it didn't involve giving up, but even that sounded too passive. For me, laughter was the only suitable response to what was coming. (198)

B36. *A Parkinson's Primer: An Indispensable Guide to Parkinson's Disease for Patients and Their Families*, by John M. Vine. Philadelphia: Paul Dry Books, 2017. xi + 154 pp.

> "It finally dawned on me that the 'Why me?' question was based on the erroneous assumption that I was entitled to an illness-free life."

When John Vine, then a sixty-year-old lawyer based in Washington, DC, was diagnosed with Parkinson's disease in 2004, he and his wife Joanne looked for a book to help them understand what the diagnosis meant. They wanted a nontechnical but reasonably comprehensive guide to his disease, where he got it, why he got it, what lay in store for them now that he had it, and what to do about it. Not finding the book he was looking for, he decided to write it. He talked to his doctors, read around in the books that were available, interviewed a score of others who had or were married to people with the disease, and put together this "primer." In his Preface he says:

> The literature on Parkinson's was voluminous. It offered more information than we could absorb at that time. We needed a primer that was written from a recently diagnosed patient's perspective. This is the book that Joanne and I needed. It is designed to get the patient—and the patient's family and friends—started. [...] I wrote this book to help Parkinson's patients become better patients, to help their relatives become better relatives, and to help their friends become better friends. (vii)

A Parkinson's Primer contains ten chapters. Most of these are fairly traditional in their presentation of material about Parkinson's. I select for particular mention here three of the chapters that will be of particular interest to newly-diagnosed patients, those patients who are in particular need of a primer.

Chapter 1, "Diagnosis," shows the wide variety in initial symptoms that have led to a diagnosis of Parkinson's disease. For John Vine himself it was sloppy handwriting and awkward typing. For Joel Havermann it was difficulty keeping the raspberries from falling off his spoon. For Learie Phillip it was an inability to shift his right foot from the brake pedal onto the gas pedal. For Cassandra Peters it was depression she at first attributed to menopause. For Pete Riehm it was a strange reaction to medicine for a urinary tract infection. For Rick Vaughn it was an inability to hold a toothbrush in his right hand. For Glenn Roberts it was lack of an arm swing. For Scott Kragie it was constipation, trouble sleeping, and reduced eye-blinking. The point here is that Parkinson's disease creeps up on us in a wide variety of ways. Often it is initially diagnosed by the patient, the family doctor, and even a neurologist as something else or, indeed, as nothing to worry about. The takeaway here is simple: there is nothing standard about Parkinson's disease: it comes as and when it will.

Chapter 2, "Why Me?", is my favorite chapter and one of the shortest. In it John Vine shows how he initially considered himself a victim of bad luck:

> I had been told that Parkinson's was a brain disorder, that its cause was unknown, that it would gradually get worse, and that there was no cure. I also had been told that the consequences of the disease were unpredictable but might include tremors, falling, impaired speech, hallucinations, delusions, dementia, and clinical depression. (12)

Why was *he* one of the very few sixty-year-olds to get this insidious disease? What had he done to deserve such punishment? After failing to find a convincing answer to this "Why me?" question, he came to the realization that the question was based on the narcissistic assumption that he was somehow special, that he deserved to be exempt from the medical troubles that afflicted other people:

> It finally dawned on me that the "Why me?" question was based on the erroneous assumption that I was entitled to an illness-free life. I ultimately recognized that I had no such entitlement. I had no reason to believe that chronic illnesses were reserved exclusively for other people. [...] I also recognized that I had been badly mistaken in viewing myself as a victim of bad luck. On the whole, my life had been blessed by good luck. (13)

What did he mean by good luck? He meant the same sorts of things that most of us can claim: he had a good family of origin and a broadening education; he had a good spouse and delightful children; he had a good job and a nice place to live; he had the good fortune to be diagnosed with Parkinson's after levodopa became available and after deep brain stimulation was approved and improved as a surgical option; he had the support of doctors, family members, and friends.

Chapter 10, "The Bell Lap," is about dying. The title is a reference to the warning bell that is rung at the start of the final lap in a long race. Its purpose is to give the competitors a warning that the race is almost over and that they should make use of the last lap to pour forth their best energies. John Vine considered that he was lucky to have been diagnosed with Parkinson's disease because it served as a warning that he was about to run the last lap:

> Like the bell at a track meet, Parkinson's tells me that there is limited time left to take care of any unfinished business. Parkinson's tells me that the finish line is not far off. [...] The less time I think I have, the more precious time seems. The more precious time seems, the more thought I give to how, and with whom, I spend it. (128–29)

John Vine is to be commended for being one of the very few of the very many who write about Parkinson's to raise the topic of death and dying, but in the end, he too steers clear of the real issues, like how people with Parkinson's are likely to die. Will it be a sudden death caused by a fall down the stairs and a broken neck or a broken hip? Will it be a long and lingering death? Will it be pneumonia? Will it be infected bedsores? If it is a long, lingering death, what is the cost and who pays for it? John Vine thinks about "how or when I will die from Parkinson's," and he is fully aware that many people say that "Parkinson's patients die *with* Parkinson's, not *from* Parkinson's." This chapter was a good opportunity for him to raise the tough questions of what might we do if we do not want to saddle our families with the personal and financial burdens of our long and lingering death. He dances around such issues, but in the end, he dances away from them: "I find it much more productive," he says, in the last sentence of the last paragraph of the last chapter of *A Parkinson's Primer*, "to focus on how I will live with Parkinson's" (130).

Shelf C: Novels in Which at Least One Character Has Parkinson's

C1. *The Distinguished Guest*, by Sue Miller. New York: Harper Perennial, 1995. 261 pp.

> "Her disease seemed for the first time a visceral thing, a tree trunk growing inside her, filling her with thickness, woodiness, and now tentacling into her thoughts, her soul itself, hardening them."

The title character in this novel is Lily Maynard, who made an unlikely name for herself when she published at age seventy-two (in 1982) her first book, her memoirs, which became a best seller and paved the way for her to become a famous writer of short stories. Her grown children, especially Alan and Clary, are both embarrassed, even annoyed, at all that she has revealed about herself, her family, and her divorce from her husband (their father) Paul, the white minister in a mostly-black Protestant church in Chicago. The novel begins when Lily comes to live with Alan and his French wife Gaby in their New England home. She needs to live with them only because she has Parkinson's and can no longer take care of herself. Her announced plan is to live as Alan and Gaby's (distinguished) guest only until a spot opens up for her in a nearby nursing home.

Very little in physical action occurs in this quiet novel until the closing pages, when a hurricane wallops the New England town. The main character, it turns out, is not so much Lily as her troubled son Alan, an

architect. His mother's visit stirs up feelings in him about his wife and their
two nearly-grown sons, Thomas and Ettie. It is gradually revealed that
both Alan and Gaby have had not-very-successful love affairs. A small plot
complication is introduced when a young woman named Linnett comes
to town for a month to act as Lily's secretary in exchange for the chance
to interview the famous Lily Maynard for an article she is writing for the
New Yorker. It seems for a time that either Thomas or Alan might develop a
romantic interest in Linnett, but nothing comes of either friendship.

My own central interest in reading this novel was in Lily Maynard
herself, her symptoms, and her death. We learn about her difficulty with
eating:

> Lily will take all morning to eat the cereal. This is what it's come
> to, Parkinson's. Worst so far is in her face, which is frozen in blank,
> childish expectancy; and in her throat, so that swallowing is a slow,
> consciously controlled activity. She has been taking the evening
> meal with Gaby and Alan, but she eats almost nothing, preferring to
> wait until she's alone again to struggle with solid food (though Gaby,
> seeing how little Lily manages to get down even then, has recently
> begun to put her dinner into the blender before she brings it in to
> Lily). (48–49)

We find other references to her face—"the blank stare of a Parkinson's face"
(92), "the frigid Parkinson's grimace" (185)—and to her tremors: "Lily set
her glass down now, and her hands, lying in her lap, moved incessantly,
a repetitive, curling, jittery motion of the fingers against the pads of her
thumbs" (176).

There is never any mention of the medications Lily takes, who gives
them to her, or how she reacts to them. There is, in sum, relatively little in
the novel about Parkinson's itself. The effects of the disease on Lily seem,
for her, to focus primarily on her declining ability to write: "Then the
Parkinson's started and it gradually grew harder for her to write. In fact, the
last two stories Lily has published were written years earlier. She revised
them a little before she sent them off, and pretended to everyone that they
were her latest productions. Privately she knew better" (50). She tries to
dictate a story to Linnett, but finally admits to her the difficulty: "I just can't
make my mind … stay on it. I want—or my *mind* wants. To go its own way.
I just stop. It's … it's Parkinson's" (95). It is finally the loss of her ability to
write that does Lily in:

> Through the long weekend, Lily had closed in on herself. She had come to understand that she was to live a life in which the words would simply be stopped. The writing, the endless long imaginative arguments about life, wouldn't be there anymore. Her disease seemed for the first time a visceral thing, a tree trunk growing inside her, filling her with thickness, woodiness, and now tentacling into her thoughts, her soul itself, hardening them. (166)

In the end, Lily's inability to write makes her want to die. In an unlikely ending she suddenly has a "good day" and is able to get up unassisted, dress herself, lie to her caretakers, mix some poison with ice cream, and swallow it. Somehow this previously incapacitated woman manages to muster enough magical self-mobility to commit suicide. But in the end, we are made to care less about the effect of her death on her than its effect on those around her.

C2. *Long, Lean, and Lethal*, by Heather Graham. Rockland, Massachusetts: Wheeler Publishing, 2000. 410 pp.

> "I've watched her suffer, I've been to the doctors, we've tried one medication and then another, and in different doses. We've dealt with tremors, choking, violent shaking, the medications, the delusions caused by the medications, and so on."

A retired actress named Abby Sawyer has Parkinson's, but she is well cared for by her loving daughter, Jennifer Sawyer, and Edgar, the butler, who has charge of her medications. Edgar describes the disease to a visitor as "horrible and cruel, dehumanizing, and she didn't deserve it" (23). The disease may be affecting Abby's thinking, though, because she becomes convinced that her daughter is being stalked by a serial killer.

To help her daughter, Abby convinces the famous actor Conar Markham, her former husband's son by a previous marriage but almost like a real son to her, to return to Los Angeles. He comes ostensibly to take a role in the soap opera that Jennifer is a star in, but really to protect Jennifer. Conar is happy to do what his loving stepmother says, even though he has never liked his stepsister Jennifer. Jennifer likes him no better and resents her mother's bringing Conar in to look after her when she feels that she is in no danger at all. The two disagree about almost everything, including whether Abby should have brain surgery for the Parkinson's.

Abby has in fact only a small role in the plot, which is complicated by the cascading bodies of more and more murdered beautiful actresses and by growing evidence that Jennifer is indeed in danger. Occasional descriptions of Abby's symptoms do enter the story: "[H]er hands were shaking more and more visibly, one with greater spasms than the other. Her head was shaking as well" (39). Jennifer at one point angrily describes to Conar what she has seen her mother go through:

> "I've been struggling with a massive downhill slide in the degeneration of her disease for almost a year. [...] I've watched her suffer, I've been to the doctors, we've tried one medication and then another, and in different doses. We've dealt with tremors, choking, violent shaking, the medications, the delusions caused by the medications, and so on." (78)

Later Jennifer glances "at the tray that held a carafe of water and her mother's medications. So many pills" (92).

We occasionally enter Abby's own mind: "Her disease often made her feel as if she were choking. As if she couldn't breathe, and couldn't swallow. She always kept a handkerchief at hand, ready to discreetly soak up any saliva she couldn't manage" (89). But usually it is the rivals Jennifer and Conar who talk about what to do. We know that Abby wants to get the vaguely-detailed "surgery"—apparently deep brain stimulation, though we are never told that. We know that the emotional Jennifer is against it because it is a very dangerous operation: " 'Conar, she could die.' " To that the sensible Conar replies, "Jennifer, she doesn't feel that she's really living. ... Jennifer, she shakes. She can maintain a normal mode of behavior for about half an hour on a truckload of medication. She won't always be eligible for surgery" (245). In the end Abby does have the surgery, which apparently works miraculously well. We last see her looking over scripts for movies in which she has been offered starring roles.

Long, Lean, and Lethal is never really about Abby, though, and its murder-mystery plot creaks to its obvious end mostly without her. Bitter rivals Jennifer and Conar, of course, do fall in love and marry. The mysterious murderer does attack Jennifer, then forces her to take a shower so he can do to her what the psychopathic murderer did to Janet Leigh in the movie *Psycho*. I won't tell you who the Hitchcock-obsessed murderer is, but just maybe the butler done it.

I do not recommend *Long, Lean, and Lethal* for plot, characterization, or information about Parkinson's. A better title might by *Long, Limp, and Lumbering*.

C3. *The Corrections*, by Jonathan Franzen. New York: Farrar, Straus, and Giroux, 2001. 568 pp.

> "These shaking hands belonged to nobody but him, and yet they refused to obey him. They were like bad children."

Retired railroad engineer Alfred Lambert has been married for nearly fifty years to his wife Enid. Their three children Gary, Chip, and Denise have all long since left their Midwestern home and have taken up fairly miserable lives of their own in the East. Financial adviser Gary lives in Philadelphia with his wife, his three sons, and his depression. Middle child Chip, having been denied tenure as an English professor and having tried unsuccessfully to write a play, accepts an unlikely job offer in politically unstable Lithuania. The youngest, Denise, lives in Philadelphia after a failed marriage and an unsuccessful affair with a married man. None of them—wife or children—knows how to deal with the stubborn Alfred's advancing Parkinson's disease.

Enid deals with the disease largely by denial. If her husband Alfred did his exercises, she thinks, he would be just fine. She seems to blame him for his own disabilities. When Alfred falls down the basement stairs carrying a box of pecans, she worries more about the pecans than about Alfred. She refuses to consider putting him in a nursing home or leaving the house they have lived in for most of their marriage. She pins her hopes on a new medicine called Correctol and pins her dreams on getting their three children home for one last Midwestern Christmas. They all finally make it home, with predictable family frictions and frustrations and guilt-giving accusations.

Alfred suffers many of the well-known symptoms of Parkinson's— imbalance, swallowing difficulties, tremors, isolation, forgetfulness, constipation, incontinence, confusion, depression, even, finally, madness. Especially effective are the descriptions of his tremors: "These shaking hands belonged to nobody but him, and yet they refused to obey him. They were like bad children. Unreasoning two-year-olds in a tantrum of selfish misery. The more sternly he gave orders, the less they listened and the more miserable and out of control they got" (67). "Alfred's hands were rotating on his wrists like the twin heads of an eggbeater" (462). Alfred has read up on his disease, but there are chapters in the Parkinson's books that he cannot bear to read: "Chapters devoted to the problems of swallowing; to the late torments of the tongue, to the final breakdown of the signal system…" (68). To avoid having to live those chapters, Alfred has purchased a shotgun and a box of shells. He makes confused plans to shoot himself in the basement: "You fitted the barrel of the shotgun into your mouth and you reached for the switch" (463). But the closest he seems to come is to give himself an enema.

Alfred never accomplishes suicide-by-shotgun, and finally his family decides to put him in a nursing home, named significantly the Deepmire Home. In his confusion—or is it his clarity?—he thinks Deepmire is a prison. He begs his favorite child Chip to help him end all the agony, but Chip, logically enough, says he cannot.

Enid visits Alfred most days at Deepmire, but has her own reason for doing so: to tell him how wrong he has been:

> He was wrong to attempt to hang himself with bedsheets in the night. He was wrong to hurl himself against the window. He was wrong to try to slash his wrist with a dinner fork. Altogether he was wrong about so many things that, except for her four days in New York and her two Christmases in Philadelphia and her three weeks in recovery from hip surgery, she never failed to visit him. She had to tell him, while she still had time, how wrong he'd been and how right she'd been. (568)

After two years at Deepmire and several failed attempts to kill himself, Alfred stops eating: "He lay curled up on the bed and barely breathed. He moved for nothing and responded to nothing except to shake his head emphatically, once, if Enid tried to put an ice chip in his mouth. The one thing he never forgot was how to refuse" (568). He escapes at last from the misery of his Parkinson's prison.

The Corrections focuses more on the family's reaction to Alfred's Parkinson's than on Alfred's Parkinson's, but in doing so it helps to convey the fact that Parkinson's is, after all, a family disease, one that, if allowed to go on too long, paralyzes everyone who has to associate with it. And it seems, like so many novels about the disease, to be sympathetic to, even if it does not actively advocate, euthanasia. Alfred wants out. *The Corrections* seems to say, "Hey, why not?"

C4. *Family Matters*, by Rohinton Mistry. New York: Vintage International (Random House), 2002. iv + 434 pp.

> "By the time Grandpa died, his back was covered with sores. Some were horrible, big and deep. Every time I looked at them, I felt a sharp pain in my back. The smell of pus and sulpha was always in the room."

Set entirely in modern-day Bombay, *Family Matters* deals with the tensions resulting from the need to care for an aging father/stepfather/grandfather when he can no longer take care of himself. Just before his seventy-ninth birthday, Nariman Vakeel, a retired English professor who has advanced Parkinson's, sprains his ankle, having ignored the advice of his stepson Jal Contractor and his stepdaughter Coomy Contractor, that he stay safely indoors. Jal and Coomy, both in their forties, have been saddled, upon the death of their mother, with the unenviable task of taking care of their recalcitrant stepfather. Their biological father, Palonji Contractor, had died of pleurisy years earlier, when they were very young. Their widowed mother, Yasmin Contractor, had then taken a second husband, Nariman Vakeel, in a marriage arranged by her parents and his. It was a first marriage for Nariman, though he had earlier had a long-term romance with Lucy Braganza, a woman whom he loved but whom he could not marry because she was of a lower caste than he. In the first year of his marriage to Yasmin, Yasmin had given birth to a lovely daughter, Roxana. Roxana eventually married Yezad Chenoy.

In a moment of King Lear-like foolish generosity, Nariman had given the large house he lived in to his two stepchildren, with the understanding that they would look after him in his old age. He had then, to keep things even, purchased and given to Roxana, his own biological daughter and her husband, a small two-room house on the other side of Bombay. Roxana and Yezad Chenoy had two sons, Murad and Jehangir, aged thirteen and nine when they come across town with their parents to celebrate their grandfather's seventy-ninth birthday. By this time Nariman owns no property and has given over to his stepchildren control of his meager pension.

Not long after his birthday, Nariman again goes out for a walk in the neighborhood, but slips into a ditch and this time breaks his ankle. The doctors at the local hospital x-ray the ankle, set it, put it in a heavy plaster cast, and then send Nariman home with instructions that he must put no weight on that leg for at least four weeks. His two stepchildren, Jal and Coomy, make a half-hearted effort to take care of him, but dealing with his rancid dentures, sloppy sponge baths, slippery bedpans, smelly in-bed bursts of diarrhea, and splashy urine bottles is too much for them. Coomy, who is especially put off by the caregiving duties, arranges to deliver Nariman to Roxana and Yezad's tiny house on the other side of Bombay.

The victim of emotional blackmail by her selfish half-sister Coomy, the generous Roxana agrees to make room for her father for a few weeks. She can do so only by making her sons sleep on the balcony in an improvised tent made of a borrowed tablecloth. Because Coomy lies to Roxana by telling her that her father's own funds had long-since given out, Roxana has almost to starve her husband and her sons to provide medicine and food for Nariman. Their situation becomes even more dire when Roxana's husband Yezad loses the small amount he has saved by gambling it away in an illegal lottery, and then loses his job when his boss is murdered and the company he had worked in for fifteen years is closed down.

The selfish Coomy, wanting to head off her stepfather's return home, persuades her older, kinder, but weaker brother Jal to knock plaster off the ceiling of Nariman's room in their house. She then lies about it to Roxana, saying that the damage had been caused by a collapsed water tank on the roof, and that it would be impossible to have Nariman come home until the damage is repaired and the ceiling is replastered. Coomy, of course, is in no rush to get the repairs made, and four months later, Nariman is still living with the impossibly impoverished and crowded Roxana, Yezad, and their sons.

Coomy finally hires an incompetent handyman-repairman to fix the plaster. She wants an incompetent handyman because she wants him to drag the work out as long as possible. He convinces her that there is a rotten beam in the ceiling. He arranges to strengthen it with a steel beam. When it turns out that the new steel beam needs a small in-place adjustment, Coomy offers to help. In the process, however, the steel beam comes crashing down and kills both the incompetent handyman and the deceitful Coomy.

Coomy's death clears the way for her brother Jal finally to take charge. He arranges for the big house to be renovated so that Nariman, Roxana,

Yezad, and their two sons can move home. He also arranges for the advantageous sale of the Chenoy's little house for enough money to let them all live comfortably.

So, where is Parkinson's in all this? It is there, but subtly. When Roxana sees her father at the birthday party, she notices that he "shuffled towards his chair" and she "wondered if her father's feet were dragging more than the last time they met; he was definitely more stooped" (20). When a retired doctor-neighbor is asked to examine Nariman after he breaks his ankle, he refuses: "Whenever your father leaves in the evening, I watch him from the window. He suffers from Parkinson's, doesn't he? [...] I could tell from the way he takes his steps" (44). Nariman himself notices a change in the way he writes: "He examined the page when he finished, curious about his wobbly handwriting. The letters grew progressively smaller from beginning to end, he hadn't been able to control their size. This was something new—another symptom of Parkinsonism, he assumed" (52). It is indeed: it is called micrographia. Later he has "troubles with his speech" (271) and has "indistinct speech" (373)—common symptoms of Parkinson's.

Although it is the broken ankle that incapacitates Nariman, it is the Parkinson's that keeps him in bed: "More than the present, the future worried Coomy. Even if Pappa's ankle mended, letting him move around a little, it wouldn't be long before he was bedridden again. Dr. Tarapore had warned that Parkinson's would incapacitate him" (147). Coomy is the most despicable character in the novel, but the real villain is Parkinson's itself, especially its unremitting and unforgiving progression: "Doctor says we cannot really hope for improvement in Parkinson's" (259). Yezad refers to "this damned Parkinson's, cruel as torture" (310). "That's the problem with the damned Parkinson's," muttered the doctor. "Never gets better" (356).

Parkinson's makes the people who have it miserable by limiting their mobility and their sense of self-worth—"I'm such a burden," Nariman says (55)—but it also dehumanizes the people whose lives it touches indirectly. Coomy has no reason to hate the stepfather who helped to raise her and who gave her a house to live in, but when he gets sick she says, "I can't help hating him" (71). Yezad loves his wife and is grateful for the house they received as a wedding present from Nariman, but when his father-in-law gets sick and moves in, Yezad lashes out at his wife: "Let me tell you, I didn't marry you for the honor and privilege of nursing your father" (206).

During Nariman's four months in the tiny house, the younger of the Chemoy sons, the nine-year-old Jehangir, bonds closely with his grandfather. He vows someday to write about his family: "Jehangir said he was going to write a big fat book when he grew up, called *The*

Complete History of the Chenoy and Vakeel Families (41). *Family Matters* is presumably that book. In the Epilogue, Jehangir emerges as the first-person narrator. He reports that five years after they had all moved back to Nariman's large home, his grandfather Nariman finally died. It was not a pleasant death:

> By the time Grandpa died, his back was covered with sores. Some were horrible, big and deep. Every time I looked at them, I felt a sharp pain in my back. The smell of pus and sulpha was always in the room. Grandpa didn't make a sound despite the agony he was going through. I wished he would scream. To see him lie quietly was more sad." (408)

C5. *Seizure*, by Robin Cook, MD. New York: G. P. Putnam's Sons, 2003. 459 pp.

> "You're allowing yourself to be experimented upon. You have no idea what the outcome may be."

A long-time U.S. Senator named Ashley Butler has long opposed, largely for his own political gain, stem-cell research. He hopes to ride his popularity among pro-life voters all the way to the presidency in the next election by sponsoring a bill that would kill the promising research program of maverick researchers like Dr. Daniel Lowell, whose work has produced remarkable cures for Parkinson's in laboratory mice.

But when Senator Butler finds himself diagnosed with Parkinson's himself, he arranges a secret meeting with Dr. Lowell, offering to let the bill die in committee if Dr. Lowell will secretly and illegally use him as the first human recipient of an attempt at a stem-cell Parkinson's cure. Although it is unethical for him to accept the bribe, Dr. Lowell is ambitious and greedy enough to accept the deal, despite Senator Butler's further condition that his experimental cell implant be tinged with blood cells taken from the Shroud of Turin.

This unlikely plot becomes impossibly complicated as Dr. Lowell and his research partner Dr. Stephanie D'Augustino, who is also his lover, fly first to Turin to acquire a bit of the bloodstained Shroud, then on to Nassau, in the Bahamas, to prepare the cells that they will surgically deposit into

Senator Butler's brain. Both in Turin and in Nassau they encounter a series of dangerous evil people and dangerous near-disasters. After surviving all of these, they finally manage to implant the properly prepared cells into Senator Butler's brain, but the lack of proper equipment in a Bahamian infertility clinic run by greedy felons leads the neurosurgeon to place the cells in the wrong place in Butler's brain. Senator Butler's Parkinson's is, apparently, cured, but he exhibits bizarre behavior and has a "seizure"— thus the title of the novel. During a second seizure a couple of days after his operation, Senator Butler seizes Dr. Lowell and leaps with him from the thirty-second floor of their Nassau hotel. They both die, victims of their own selfish and unethical pride.

Readers are hard put to like anyone in this novel. Dr. Stephanie D'Augustino has some good instincts but little backbone, and she too easily goes along with the doomed plans of her lover. Dr. Lowell lacks moral backbone and is blinded by his own dreams for a Nobel prize. Senator Butler has backbone but no sense of right and wrong. His administrative assistant Carol Manning is not a bad person, but she is more interested in her own political future as Butler's successor in the Senate than in helping him. Readers of the novel who have Parkinson's may feel some sympathy for Senator Butler. Carol warns him that "You're allowing yourself to be experimented upon. You have no idea what the outcome may be," Butler ignores her warning:

> "It may be true that I do not know the outcome for sure, but it is
> also true that if I were to do nothing in the face of my progressive,
> otherwise incurable neurological degenerative disease, I know
> exactly what the outcome would be. My daddy preached that the
> Good Lord helps those who help themselves. All my life I have been
> a fighter, and I am not going to stop now. I am not going out with
> a whimper. I will be kicking and screaming like a bagged polecat."
> (109)

Bagged by his seizure and screaming obscenities, he does just that. Surely some people with Parkinson's would consider allowing themselves to be experimented upon for a chance at a promising cure. Even if they died doing so, their death might have bolstered the possibilities of finding a cure for others. Surely some would feel that a kicking and screaming death is better than the long slow freezing of the alternative.

In the end, the two women head off into the horizon, Dr. D'Augustino to continue the search for the cure that Dr. Lowell had envisioned, Carol to a Senate seat from which she would help researchers do their science without political interference. Meanwhile, the real hero of this story is the CURE itself, the cure that strives to free itself from its political and scientific chains. Author Robin Cook has a degree in medicine and openly advocates, both in the novel itself and in a polemical Author's Note at the end, that politicians must not meddle with ongoing scientific research. While politicians play their vote-winning games, he says, people who might otherwise be cured suffer and die.

C6. *Blackbelly*, by Heather Sharfeddin. Bridgehampton, New York: Bridge Works Publishing, 2005. 240 pp.

> "As he looked at his father, he made a firm decision to kill himself before he wound up like that. He wondered if his father would've committed suicide if it hadn't been for his faith."

The Parkinson's victim in this silly novel is brought home to die by his forty-something unmarried son, a modern-day shepherd, who hates his father but wants him to die at home rather than in a nursing home. To make it possible for his father to come home, Chas McPherson hires a drug-addicted nurse named Mattie Holden to live in his Idaho ranch home and take care of the old man, usually identified merely as Mr. McPherson. Mr. McPherson had once been the fiercely sin-oriented town preacher, but now he is in the "late stages" of Parkinson's: "He doesn't talk. Doesn't walk. Barely eats" (6). In contemplating the job offer, Mattie is familiar enough with the disease to know that Mr. McPherson will be "incapable of even the most basic tasks. He'd need feeding, diapering, bathing, massage. She promised to do her best in making this man's last days comfortable" (8–9).

Mr. McPherson is pathetic in his immobility: he never says anything, never touches anything, seems never to notice anything that goes on around him. In his catatonic state he serves merely to be the means of bringing Chas and Mattie together and of providing Mattie with an unresponsive audience for her occasional self-revealing monologues.

Yes, of course Chas and Mattie fall in love. When Mr. McPherson's disease has served its purpose of causing Chas and Mattie to live under the same roof, he conveniently dies—but not before making his son contemplate suicide: "As he looked at his father, he made a firm decision to kill himself before he wound up like that. He wondered if his father would've committed suicide if it hadn't been for his faith. Probably he would have—probably had to struggle not to. He'd once been a powerful man, physically as well as mentally" (130). The novel seems almost to endorse suicide or euthanasia for people with Parkinson's.

There are some minor characters like a Muslim family whose house is burned down by an arsonist and a genial sheriff who for a while considers Chas McPherson to be a suspect, but nothing much is made of them. It is troubling in that the book lacks evidence that the author knows or wants to know much about Parkinson's. The jacket blurb says that author Heather Sharfeddin and her husband raise blackbellies on their ranch in Oregon. "Blackbellies" are a species of hairy, as opposed to wooly, sheep that Chas McPherson raises on his ranch. Clearly, Sharfeddin understands more about blackbellies than she does about Parkinson's.

Old Mr. McPherson never comes alive as a character. We are never given any reason to like him or to care about him. Indeed, it would be easy enough to surmise that the author wants us to see his Parkinson's as just punishment for his nasty ways as a younger man. His parental rigidity as a father and his moral rigidity as a preacher are punished by his physical rigidity as a Parkinson's victim. In any case, we are given little reason to sympathize with him or to be sad when he dies.

C7. *Suspect*, by Michael Robotham. New York: Vintage, 2005. 353 pp.

> "This disease is like a distant train, hurtling through the darkness toward us. It might seem like a long way off, but it's coming."

Joseph O'Loughlin, the narrator of *Suspect*, a practicing clinical psychologist and part-time professor at Bath University in the UK, has Parkinson's. As if that is not trouble enough, he gets caught up in a web of murders. As he tries to help the police identify a corpse by using his skills as a psychologist to discover her identity and to determine what kind of man would commit such an awful murder, he suddenly finds himself to be a prime suspect. Soon there are more murders, and Joe runs, not only from Detective Inspector Vincent Ruiz of the London police corps but also from Bobby Morgan, a psychotic patient of his who wants to frame him for the

murders and wants him to die a miserable death—but not before Bobby
kills some more people. The plot is too complex to review here, but it all
comes out more or less okay in the end—after Joe's wife and daughter, and
Joe himself, are almost killed.

Joe O'Loughlin is forty-two years old when his friend and doctor, Jock,
gives him the Parkinson's diagnosis. Many of his symptoms sound so
accurate that I at first found myself thinking that Robotham himself must
have the disease. He seems to be speaking from the inside:

> If it's early in the week and I'm rested, I will have just a little trouble
> getting the fingers of my left hand to cooperate. Buttons will find
> buttonholes, belts will find belt loops, and I can even tie a Windsor
> knot. On my bad days, such as this one, it is a different story. The
> man I see in the mirror will need two hands to shave and will arrive
> at the breakfast table with bits of toilet paper stuck to his neck and
> chin. (11)

> My left arm is trembling and I grasp the back of a chair to keep my
> hands steady. (14)

> I sit and force my hand between my knees to stop the tremors. (160)

> I start typing an e-mail using my right hand, pressing one key at a
> time. I tuck my left hand under my thigh to stop it trembling. (320)

There are some really good lines in *Suspect*:

> Nobody ever dies of Parkinson's disease. You die with it. That's
> one of Jock's trite aphorisms. I can just see it on a bumper sticker
> because it's only half as ridiculous as "Guns don't kill people,
> people do." (49)

> This disease is like a distant train, hurtling through the darkness
> toward us. It might seem like a long way off, but it's coming. (52)

> I am losing my body bit by bit. Slowly it is abandoning me. (98)

> I know it will get worse. But what the hell! I'm lucky. A lot of
> people have Parkinson's. Not all of them have a beautiful wife, a
> loving daughter and a new baby to look forward to. (353)

Some of the descriptions, however, sound suspiciously as if they came from a medical textbook, especially those that emanate from Jock:

> "Sometimes when I try to get out of a chair or of bed, my mind says get up but nothing happens." [...] "That's called starting hesitancy." (47)

> There are no diagnostic tests for Parkinson's. An experienced neurologist relies on observation, looking for the tremors, stiffness, impaired balance, and slowness of movement. The disease is chronic and progressive. It is not contagious, nor is it usually inherited. (50)

> He's talking about the Parkinson's mask. Jock had warned me of the possibility. My face can become totally unresponsive and expressionless like an Easter Island statue. (85)

> "Stem-cell research is going to provide a breakthrough," he adds, sounding upbeat. "In five or ten years they'll have a cure." (87)

> "What about exercise?" "It can help, according to Jock, but it won't stop the disease." (100)

> I sit on the toilet. My nerves have me constipated or maybe it's the medication. (154)

> The bradykinesia is becoming more obvious. Stress is a factor in Parkinson's disease. (181).

There are other problems with Robotham's portrayal of Parkinson's. All of Joe's symptoms seem to be conflated, rushed together, whereas for most patients they are progressive, developing one at a time, over time. In just a few weeks after diagnosis, however, Joe has them all: tremor, freezing, bradykinesia, constipation, and so on. Some of those typically take years to develop. Also, he moves too quickly in his medications from selegiline to levodopa. And then there is the smell thing: "I have never been able to work out why herbal tea smells so wonderful" (230), Joe says at one point. In fact, however, most people with Parkinson's people can't smell much at all, not even the bold odors of their own bodies, let alone the subtle aromas of herbal teas.

Finally, it does not sound right to me that Joe goes to a hooker right after he is diagnosed: "On the same day I learn of my progressive neurological disease I sleep with another woman—getting my fill of sex and excitement before my body falls apart" (174). That does not sound convincing to me. The last thing I wanted to do the day I was diagnosed was locate a hooker. Angry, self-pitying, confused, and frightened, I went home with Anne. That's where my comfort lay.

C8. *Lost*, by Michael Robotham. New York: Mulholland Books (Little, Brown), 2005. 395 pp.

> "How's the Parkinson's?"
> Joe replies, "I've stopped ordering soup at restaurants."

Joe O'Loughlin appears in *Lost*, but only in a cameo role. The main character in this novel is Detective Inspector Ruiz. The story opens with Ruiz, wounded and nearly dead from loss of blood and hypothermia, being dragged from the Thames. Because he has situational amnesia, he has no idea who shot him or why, how he wound up in the icy waters of the Thames, whether he shot anyone in the process of getting himself shot, or who tries to murder him as he lies recuperating in the hospital. With the help of his friend Joe O'Loughlin, he tries to reconstruct the events from the fragmentary hints he gets from others. When asked if he has the diamonds, he has no idea what diamonds are being referred to. When he is asked about who were the two others whose blood, besides his own—blood the police had found on the boat drifting downriver where their bodies are now—he has no recollection of any boat or any bodies. When asked why he had the previous day talked about Mickey, the little girl who disappeared three years earlier, as if she might still be alive, he does not know how to answer, since he recalls only how he had helped convince a jury back then that Mickey had been murdered by a man who was now in prison for the crime.

Joe's role in this complicated plot is minor, but he helps Ruiz come to terms with feeling guilty for his role in a toboggan accident many years earlier, and in doing so helps Ruiz to solve the mystery of the "lost" Mickey. We still find references to Joe's Parkinson's disease: Joe makes little jokes about his disease. He tells Ruiz, for example, that he likes his martinis shaken, not stirred. When Ruiz asks him "How's the Parkinson's?" Joe replies, "I've stopped ordering soup at restaurants" (29). At one point the narrator Ruiz remarks that Joe seemed to be "unaware of his twitches and trembles" (69). Later Ruiz remarks that Parkinson's "will rob [Joe] of old age" (185). As in *Suspect*, however, in *Lost* the Parkinson's is an overlay and does not in itself influence the plot.

C9. *Shatter*, by Michael Robotham. New York: Mulholland Books (Little, Brown), 2008. 472 pp.

> "There's a third person in our marriage. His name is Mr. Parkinson and he took up residence four years ago."

Professor Joe O'Loughlin finds the police waiting for him as he leaves his lecture to a class of psychology students at Bath University. The police tell him that they want him to come with them immediately to "talk down" a blonde, apparently in her forties, naked except for her red shoes. She is standing outside the safety barrier on a bridge, apparently ready to jump. No one knows who she is or why she wants to commit suicide. Joe rushes to the bridge and tries to talk the woman into coming back to safety, but he discovers that she is listening intently to someone else on a cell phone, someone who seems to give her competing advice. Joe watches the blonde woman step off the bridge and plummet to her death.

It is relatively easy to discover the identity of the naked woman. The police find her car parked not far from the bridge and soon determine that the dead woman is named Christine Wheeler. She had left no suicide note, and no one can figure out why she jumped. The police cannot retrieve the cell phone from the bottom of the river and they have no idea who Christine had been talking to on the phone. Then a sixteen-year-old woman named Darcy Wheeler shows up and announces that the dead woman was her mother and that her mother did not commit suicide but must have been murdered: "The police say it was suicide but that's impossible. Mum wouldn't … she couldn't. Not like that. […] Mum hated heights. I mean really hated them" (48, 50).

The police, led by Detective Inspector Veronica Cray, refuse to take seriously Darcy's insistence that her mother had been murdered. They ignore her until they are confronted by the apparent suicide of Christine's friend and business partner, Sylvia Furness. Sylvia's body, naked except for her pointy-toed black boots, is found suspended by handcuffs from a tree. In the mud at her feet is found an untraceable cell phone. Joe believes that Christine and Sylvia were indeed murdered. He calls on his friend

Vincent Ruiz, a retired police detective, to help him discover the identity, the methods, and the whereabouts of the murderer, who turns out to be a deranged AWOL army officer named Gideon Tyler. They discover that the British army is eager to locate and arrest Gideon, who knew top-secret information about methods of surveillance and torture. Gideon is very clever, however, and has eluded both the military and the municipal police efforts to find him. Gideon's motives in murdering the two women are never fully revealed, but we come to understand that Christine and Sylvia had both been classmates of Helen Tyler, the woman Gideon had married but who had run off with their daughter Chloe. Helen and Chloe had both been reported drowned when the Greek ferry they were traveling on capsized. Gideon has convinced himself, however, that his wife and daughter are both still alive, and hopes that the deaths of Helen's two classmates will bring his wife and daughter out of hiding.

Joe's life gets dangerously complicated when Gideon manages to abduct both his lovely wife Julianne and his older daughter Charlotte (who goes by the nickname "Charlie"). There is no need for me to reveal here the methods by which Joe captures the evil Gideon and locates Julianne and Charlie. And it is not necessary that I review the unlikely series of events that lead Joe to accuse his wife of infidelity and lead her to abandon their marriage. I should mention, however, that a small measure of sympathy for Gideon is generated when we learn through italicized entries into his mind that he had been routinely beaten as a young boy by his father. And, of course, I should mention the role that Parkinson's plays in *Shatter*.

In this novel Joe is forty-five years old and has lived with Parkinson's disease for four years:

> It is four years since my left hand gave me the message. It wasn't written down, or typed or printed on fancy paper. It was an unconscious, random flicker of my fingers, a twitch, a ghost movement, a shadow made real. Unknown to me then, working in secret, my brain had begun divorcing my mind. It has been a long-drawn-out separation with no legal argument over division of assets—who gets the CD collection and Aunt Grace's antique sideboard? The divorce began with my left hand and spread to my arm and my leg and my head. Now it feels as if my body is being owned and operated by someone else who looks like me. (29)

Joe has a lot to say in *Shatter* about his disease. He emphasizes the shaking (see pages 7, 15, 282, 334). He speaks of the Parkinson's "mask" (see page 19). He has trouble walking and talking at the same time (120). He now uses a cane most of the time (159, 286). He can't keep himself from rubbing his thumb and forefinger together in an inadvertent activity he calls "pill rolling" (97, 143, 286). He speaks of the panic he feels when he discovers that his daughter has been abducted:

> My arm is shaking. My leg. My chest, My head. I take a step and almost collapse, I take another and fall. I try to get up, I can't. [...] Climbing Mill Hill my left leg suddenly locks as it swings forward and I land on my face. I don't feel the pain. Dragging myself onto my feet, I start running again with a strange, stumbling goosestep. (363–64)

He talks more about the pills he needs to take (29, 82) and what happens when he does not have them at his disposal:

> There is a stale, unsavory smell in my lungs. It's coming from me. My medication has switched off suddenly. My head, shoulders and arms are writhing and jerking like a snake.
> "Are you OK?" asks Monk.
> "I need my pills."
> "Where are they?"
> "Upstairs, beside my bed. The white plastic bottle." (374)

Perhaps most interesting is Joe's speaking of his disease as a person he names "Mr. Parkinson," an intrusive and unwelcome guest whom he can blame, can hold responsible for the nastier consequences of his disease:

> Mr. Parkinson is to blame. (31)

> There are moments, I know them well, when Mr. Parkinson refuses to lie down and take his medicine like a man. He plays cruel tricks on me and embarrasses me in public. (91)

> There's a third person in our marriage. His name is Mr. Parkinson and he took up residence four years ago. (126)

> Julianne used to love my sense of fairness and compassion and my hatred of hypocrisy. Now she treats me like I have no other role to

play except to raise my children, perform a handful of lectures and wait for Mr. Parkinson to steal what he hasn't already taken. (171)

Most distressing to Joe is what this Mr. Parkinson is doing to his marriage to his beloved Julianne. To defend her decision to leave him, she tells Joe what it is like to be married to him now:

> "I don't know you anymore, Joe. You're sad. You're so, so sad. And you carry it around with you or it hangs over you like a cloud, infecting everyone around you."
>
> "I'm not sad."
>
> "You are. You worry about your disease. You worry about me. You worry about the girls. That's why you're sad. You think you're the same man, Joe, but it's not true. You don't trust people any more. You don't warm to them or go out of your way to meet them. You don't have any friends."
>
> "Yes I do." [...]
>
> "For such a clever man, how do you manage to be so stupid and self-absorbed? I've seen what you do, Joe. I've seen how you study yourself every day, looking for signs, imagining them. You want to blame someone for your Parkinson's, but there's nobody to blame. It just happened." (348)

Joe O'Loughlin is not alone. Like the rest of us, he tries to figure out who or what is to blame for the unexplained and undeservedly nasty things that happen to him.

C10. *A Good Death*, by Gil Courtemanche, translated from the French by Wayne Grady. Vancouver: Douglas and McIntyre, 2009. 207 pp.

> "He knows how to walk and talk, he's conscious, he understands everything. But he falls down, or he babbles like a baby."

The narrator of this novel has never much liked, let alone loved, his aging father, who now has what is called "rigid Parkinson's." Here is what the doctor told him:

> "It's called rigid Parkinson's, plus there's his recent stroke. I'll spare you the scientific details; let's just say there's been a communication breakdown among his neurons. The brain gives the order to walk, but the neurons don't receive the command in time and so the patient falls down. The patient wants to talk, but his vocal cords and mouth react too late. They don't receive the electric impulses soon enough. He knows how to walk and talk, he's conscious, he understands everything. But he falls down, or he babbles like a baby, and you get the feeling he isn't there and doesn't hear you. It's not that complicated. ... I forgot to mention, it's a degenerative disease." (1–2)

The man with Parkinson's is given no name. He is identified only as "my father" by the narrator, one of a number of children that "my father" and "my mother" raised. The narrator, now a sixty-year-old a playwright, has few good memories of his tyrannical father. He is repulsed by his father's gross eating habits: his father gorges himself on food, spills some of it, dirties "my mother's spotless tablecloth" (4). The narrator tells us in many ways that he does not love his father:

> Nothing makes sense to him anymore. He has words, he has thoughts, but no one hears them. He knows how to move his feet and hands, but he falls down or drops his glass. And so I sit to his left every family meal, trying to anticipate his rages and his defeats. I prefer the rages. They tell me that the man I once knew, the man I do not love, still exists. (3)

Indeed, he wishes his father were dead, if only so that his mother, who is growing more and more defeated and diminished taking care of her husband, can recover.

The plot, which takes place mostly through flashbacks and around family dinners in the holiday season, reveals the reactions of the various children to their father's condition. Some want him to live, some wish he would die, some want to kill him. The major suspense in the novel turns on when and how the corpulent, repulsive, nasty man with Parkinson's will die. Will he choke on his food? Will one of his children murder him? Will he commit suicide? We don't find the answer until the final page.

The author, who lives in Montreal, seems to have done some basic research about Parkinson's, but has little fundamental understanding of the disease and little sympathy for those who have it. One gets the feeling, at times, that he sees the disease as a fitting punishment for the father, a man who spent most of his life being unpleasant, insulting, and oppressive to his wife and children.

C11. *Bleed for Me*, by Michael Robotham. New York: Mulholland Books (Little, Brown), 2010. 419 pp.

> "What sort of wife abandons her husband when he's sick? I know that's what people are saying behind my back. I'm a hard-hearted bitch. I'm the villain."

B *leed for Me* opens with a twelve-year-old school girl cutting her own flesh so that she bleeds. She puts it this way in her diary:

> *i don't cut often. sometimes once a week, once a month. [...] once or twice i've cut too deeply but each time i managed to fix myself, using a needle and thread. i bet that makes you shudder but it didn't hurt so much and i boiled the needle first. [...] you want to know the reason? you want to know why someone would bleed in secret? it's because i deserve it. i deserve to be punished. [...] every drop removes the poison inside me, running down my arms, dripping off my fingers.* (3–4)

The writer of that diary is Sienna Hegarty, who is fourteen when the main action of the novel takes place, two years after she wrote that entry. Sienna's older sister Zoe Hegarty had been routinely sexually abused by their father, Ray Hegarty, but when a deranged fellow-student had attacked Zoe so violently that she had been consigned permanently in a wheelchair, their father begins to turn his lustful attention to Sienna. Sienna, meanwhile, has developed a crush on her high school drama teacher, Gordon Ellis. It is a crush that Ellis flirtatiously encourages, though he is careful to do so surreptitiously because he knows that it is both unethical and illegal for a teacher to have a sexual relationship with a fourteen-year-old student. Besides, Gordon is married to a young woman named Natasha, who had once been one of his students. He had married her after his first wife had mysteriously disappeared—apparently murdered by him. Sienna's life is complicated by the fact that she becomes pregnant, though she loses the fetus very early in the pregnancy.

The psychologist Joe O'Loughlin, now forty-nine, gets involved when Ray Hegarty, Sienna and Zoe's father, is found dead in his own home, his throat cut with a sharp knife. Sienna is the natural suspect, since she knew about cutting with sharp knives, first found the body, and was known to fear and distrust her father. The police, led by Detective Chief Inspector Veronica Cray, take Sienna into custody. Joe becomes involved because he knows Sienna somewhat since she was his daughter Charlie's best friend. He also knows something about Gordon Ellis, because both Sienna and Charlie are in rehearsal for the school musical, directed by Ellis. Joe thinks Sienna is innocent and he distrusts the sleazy Gordon Ellis. He soon finds himself embroiled in a viper's tangle of illicit sex, prostitution, corruption, immigration, abuse, torture, and murder.

Joe calls in his sidekick, the retired policeman Vincent Ruiz. Before the tale is done, Joe has a brief sexual encounter with Annie Robinson, the school counselor, tries unsuccessfully to patch up his marriage to the lovely Julianne, is arrested on suspicion of murder himself, and is stabbed (but not quite killed) by a knife-wielding assailant in a supermarket. It is not until the epilogue that we find out who had really killed Ray Hegarty and why. Hint: it was not Sienna or Gordon Ellis.

We find in *Bleed for Me* a number of references to Joe's Parkinson's disease. He emphasizes, for example, the fact that the disease robs him of his autonomy:

> Sometimes my legs don't do as they're told. My brain sends the messages but they fail to arrive or like London buses they come all at once causing my limbs to either lock up or take me backwards,

sideways and occasionally forwards, so that I look like I'm being operated via remote control by a demented toddler. (7)

I muster a nervous smile. At least I hope I'm smiling. That's one of the problems with my "condition." I can never be sure what face I'm showing the world—the genial O'Loughlin smile or the bland Parkinson's mask. (18)

My head and arms begin jerking uncontrollably. My medication has worn off and Mr. Parkinson, a cruel puppeteer, is tugging at my strings and twisting my body into inhuman shapes. (244)

He talks about the trouble he has with toileting:

My bladder won't do as it's told. I stand and stare at the wall. […] Nothing is happening. The queue is getting longer. […] That's one of the problems with my medication. I used to piss like a racehorse. Now I squirt and dribble. (135)

Swinging my legs over the side of the bed, my feet argue for a moment, curling inwards and not wanting to press flat on the rug. I have to concentrate, forcing my toes to the floor, then my heels. Slowly the spasms ease and I can reach the bathroom. (175)

He gives us a glimpse of what it like to be the wife of a man with Parkinson's, when he tries to win Julianna back:

"Let me come back."
She shakes her head. "I'm not strong enough to live with you, Joe. I'm barely strong enough to live without you."
"Why?"
"Because you're not always going to be here." (147)

"I don't need you to make me feel guilty. I feel guilty enough already. What sort of wife abandons her husband when he's sick? I know that's what people are saying behind my back. I'm a hard-hearted bitch. I'm the villain." (303)

And for the first time, Joe thinks seriously about his own death. Some of the references to death are subtle, like this to waking up in the morning after a night without his medications:

> My left leg and arm are twitching. Using my right hand, I pick up a small white pill and take a sip of water, raising my head from the pillow to swallow. The blue pill comes next. After twenty minutes I take another inventory. The twitches have gone and Mr. Parkinson has been kept at bay for another few hours. Never vanquished. Till death us do part. (71)

Some are more direct, as when Joe tells about his patient who invited his friends to a pub, bought them all drinks, left a note, and slipped out and drowned himself in the Thames. The note read:

> I didn't like the thought of spending my last years lying in bed, surrounded by my children and grandchildren feeling they must sit by my old wretched body until my last gasp. So I hope you'll understand and raise a glass and give me a cheer for catching the tide tonight.
>
> There's something noble about an exit like that, but I doubt I'll have the courage or the conviction. (266)

Joe returns in the epilogue to the subject of his own death: "I'd rather a mundane end than a gloriously brave or stupid one. In the meantime, I am going to tremble and twitch and spasm into middle age" (418). But Robotham is not ready to let Joe O'Loughlin die just yet. He has more work for this psychologist-professor with Parkinson's.

C12. *The Map of True Places*, by Brunonia Barry. New York: HarperCollins, 2010. 403 pp.

> "He doesn't want to live with end-stage Parkinson's," Melville said to her. "He doesn't want to wind up in a nursing home in the fetal position for the next ten years." Zee sat silently for a few minutes. "Well, he's not going to kill himself," she said finally. "Not on my watch."

The central character of *The Map of True Places* is a young psychiatrist named Zee Finch. "Zee" is short for Hepzibah. She was named for Hepzibah Pyncheon, a central character in Nathaniel Hawthorne's 1851 novel *The House of the Seven Gables*. She was given the name by her father, Finch, an American literature professor in a college in Boston who had specialized in nineteenth-century novelists. Retired and in his late sixties when the present action of *The Map of True Places* is set, he lives in Salem across the street from the famous tourist attraction, *The House of the Seven Gables*. He has recently published a book suggesting that there was an "intimate" relationship between Nathaniel Hawthorne and Herman Melville. Finch has lived with his longtime companion, Charles Thompson, whom he had nicknamed "Melville," a name everyone knows him by now. Finch suffers from late-stage Parkinson's, which manifests itself in medicine-induced hallucinations. At times, for example, he thinks he is Nathaniel Hawthorne.

The meaning of the title, *The Map of True Places*, is one of several small mysteries of the novel. There are others. What was Zee's middle name? Why had Libby Braedon, one of Zee's psychiatric patients, committed suicide by leaping off a bridge in Boston? Why had Zee's mother, Maureen Finch, when Zee was thirteen, committed suicide by swallowing strychnine? What is the relevance of the story "The Once" that Maureen Finch had written about the unhappy life of a beautiful woman named Zylphia who became the miserable wife of a sea captain named Arlis Browne? Why had Finch suddenly banished from his home his long-time companion and lover, Melville? Who will Zee marry, her fiancé Michael or the strangely attractive man named Adam, who had had a dangerous affair with Lilly Braedon and was apparently responsible for her suicide? Who was really the biological father of Zee Finch? I cannot discuss here all of these mysteries. They are all more or less resolved by the end. But there is

one mystery that I do want to discuss: how are the caregivers to respond
to the needs and desires of a man with hopeless, debilitating, late-stage
Parkinson's?

Author Brunonia Barry has apparently found a way to learn a lot about
Parkinson's disease. She peppers her descriptions of Finch with statements
like these:

> Somewhere in the distance, he could hear a phone ringing. He was
> not well today. It was not simply his knees. His head was foggy,
> more foggy than usual. And his hands had a rigidity he could not
> soften. [...] He had turned to stone, and all he could do was wait for
> the medicine or for some force of nature to release him. (57)

> Finch practiced touching his thumb to his middle finger as rapidly
> and accurately as he could. He had succeeded fairly well with his
> right hand but was slower and clumsier with his left. (63)

> His face was masked, a classic sign of Parkinson's. (64)

> He couldn't swallow very well any more. [...] Bowel movements
> were becoming increasingly difficult. (82)

> A long string of saliva dripped out of his open mouth and onto his
> pressed shirt. (83)

Zee learns that Finch is incontinent and has to wear Depends. When she
takes her father out for coffee, he tells her that he has to go to the bathroom.
She takes him into the ladies' room and guides him into a stall, then waits
outside the stall:

> She stayed, leaning against the door for what seemed a long time.
> After several more minutes, she let the door open slightly and peered
> into the stall. Finch sat, pants around his ankles, looking as if he
> were about to cry. The diaper he'd been wearing was now half on,
> half off and hanging into the toilet. [...] She gathered up the soiled
> diaper and stuffed it into the box marked Feminine Hygiene. She
> wiped him clean and helped him pull up his pants. "We'll get you a
> shower when we get home," she said. (127)

At one point Zee attends a caregiver-support meeting at a Salem hospital.

She hears the moderator's statement that "Caring for an ailing parent is a lot like caring for a baby. Except that with a baby, you get to look forward to the results" (216–17). Not long after that, she takes Finch to see his neurologist. He asks her a question:

> "How long has it been since he was diagnosed?"
> She was appalled that the doctor didn't know.
> "About ten years," she said.
> The doctor was quiet for a moment and then said in a serious but far too casual tone, "Ten years is a good long run for Parkinson's." (294)

Finch hears the doctor's pronouncement. On the way home in the car, he says to Zee, "So what he was saying is that I'm going to die soon":

> "That doctor is a son of a bitch," she said. She was about to tell him they would never go back, that neurologists were a dime a dozen in Boston, and that she'd have a new one for him by morning. But Finch spoke before she could form the words.
> "It's all right," he said. "I want to die." (295)

Finch's long-term partner Melville has meanwhile noticed that his beloved Finch has been gradually losing ground to Parkinson's and, like many other victims of the disease, has been showing signs of dementia:

> Parkinson's patients, if they lived long enough with the disease, often got what was called the "Alzheimer's crossover" and started to show signs of dementia. […] Parkinson's was one of the cruelest diseases out there. If you lived long enough with it, if something else didn't get you first, you'd end up in the fetal position in bed in some institution, sometimes for years. Melville often wondered— often hoped, in fact—that he would have the strength it took to help Finch end things if it came to that. He knew Finch's wishes, and he also knew that Finch had been saving pills for years against the inevitable. (177)

Melville has a conversation with Zee later on about her father:

> "I'm afraid he might be suicidal," she said.
> He understood. He knew that Finch didn't want to live with

the progression of the disease. But in all their conversations about the future, they had both been keenly aware of the effect any such disclosure might have on Zee.

Melville's lack of surprise shocked her. "You're not okay with it?"

"He doesn't want to live with end-stage Parkinson's," Melville said to her. "He doesn't want to wind up in a nursing home in the fetal position for the next ten years."

Zee sat silently for a few minutes. "Well, he's not going to kill himself," she said finally. "Not on my watch." (298)

Not long after that, Finch takes a bad fall, bangs his head, and breaks two ribs. He is taken to a nursing home. Zee has her way. The demented shell who was once her father, who wants to die, who no longer recognizes his daughter or his long-term partner, is kept alive in the nursing home. Sometime later, Zee and Melville go to visit him in the nursing home:

He didn't know her name any more. Didn't know Melville either. He thought that Melville was someone who worked at the nursing home, someone who came to read to him every afternoon. [...] Finch hadn't been able to use his walker again; he was in a wheelchair permanently now. (398)

Score: Zee one. Finch zero.

C13. *My Life with Belle,* by Judith Ravenscroft. London: Lenz Books, 2010. 90 pp.

> "I lived a life of extreme regularity, dictated by the timing of the medication I took. In one sense the pills, having to remember to take them, exerted a tyranny that never allowed me to forget I was sick, but mainly, as tools of control, they liberated me."

My *Life with Belle* is a confusing little novel. Its narrator is an unnamed woman with Parkinson's disease who reads the novel *Adolphe* by Benjamin Constant. The main character in that early-nineteenth-century French novel is named Ellénore, a middle-aged woman seduced by a much younger man. Apparently Constant had based his novel on the story of Isabelle de Charrière, the Belle referred to in the title of Judith Ravenscroft's novel. Belle had died in 1805. For reasons that are not entirely clear, the narrator of *My Life with Belle* decides that she is going to retell Belle's story but give it a different ending. She soon gets her own life—that of a modern-day London housewife and book editor—mixed up and confused with Belle's story. It turns out that *My Life with Belle* is confusing in large part because its narrator is experiencing the dementia that sometimes accompanies Parkinson's disease.

The narrator tells us about the early symptoms of her disease. Most of these symptoms show up when she is out walking. In her first paragraph she reports seeing "on a morning walk" what she calls an apparition: "a black-clad figure emerged from the gloom and bore down on me, pressing forward like the masthead of a noble ship. His face was blank—skin and bones, empty of personality—and he had a doomlike air" (7). In her second paragraph she reports that as she walked into town a couple of months later she "started to topple over, as if unbalanced by a tug from behind. Returning to consciousness, I was able to right myself" (7). She reports several other disturbing troubles connected to her walking:

> My back ached after such a long walk, my legs were tired. (21)

> My back almost stopped me going with friends on a long walk across the Heath. [...] A friend lagged behind with me and asked what it was, this bad back, as if he didn't quite believe in it, it didn't

correspond to what he knew of bad backs. "And you're walking oddly," he said. (23)

And what with one thing and another I fell over, tripped, and couldn't save myself, or lost my balance—afterwards I couldn't reconstruct the circumstances, but remembered the cracking sound of bone on concrete as my knees hit the floor. (24)

The narrator finally goes to a doctor who examines her and gives her the diagnosis—that she has what he calls "the malady of Doctor P." (29). The narrator goes to the library and reads the 1817 essay in which Dr. James Parkinson first described the disease that eventually was named for him: "It made harrowing reading, and I got no further than page four ('it's last stage... the wished-for release') before fleeing" (31).

She is not pleased with the diagnosis:

It seemed to me that I had crossed a border I could never traverse again, between health and sickness, autonomy and dependence, life and death. [...] I felt trapped, trapped by an illness that would soon make me dependent, trapped by the man I was dependent on, trapped not least by my lack of means. (49)

She adapts as well as she can to "the malady of Doctor P." by taking the pills that both free her and enslave her:

I lived a life of extreme regularity, dictated by the timing of the medication I took. In one sense the pills, having to remember to take them, exerted a tyranny that never allowed me to forget I was sick, but mainly, as tools of control, they liberated me. So long as I remembered to take them at exactly the right time, for much of the day I was fit and active—and if I forgot or they failed to kick in I just sat at home until they took effect. (66)

The narrator works on her Belle story but is in no hurry to finish it because she fears that doing so will finish her own life:

I've still things to write about Belle, my companion through these years of Doctor P., but I keep putting off the moment when I might finish. [...] I've put it off [...] because to write The End would be to invite my own. Now it may be too late, this malady has dried up my juices; and when I look at these fragments of writing I see a mind that is stuck. This stuckness has become the chief attribute of my condition. (85)

In *My Life with Belle*, Judith Ravenscroft has tried to show the tangled workings of the mind of a woman with Parkinson's. If we are confused by what she says, that is because her disease makes her understand things and describe things in confusing ways. Near the end, the narrator speaks of writing as "moving paragraphs around on a computer on my lap, stiffly, haltingly tapping out words which mostly I then discard—is this writing?" (85). I fear that most readers will think not. The novel does indeed read at times as if the paragraphs and chapters were dropped in almost at random.

It is time, however, for me to make an end of my little review of this little novel that will give most readers a little enlightenment but very little enjoyment.

C14. *The Diver*, by Alfred Neven DuMont, translated from the German by David Dollenmayer. New York: St. Martin's Press, 2010. 213 pp.

> "But, darling, why didn't you call me? How was I to know you were getting ready for bed so early today? How many times have I told you I'm happy to help? You need me!"

The central character in *The Diver* is an old man named Albert, now in his early eighties. He is married, still, to a woman named Ann, but gradually comes to understand, by a roundabout trail, that he had never much loved her. That trail takes him on an emotional journey that involves their daughter Gloria, Gloria's best friend Christie, and Christie's adoptive mother Lena.

Gloria is a troubled young woman who is afflicted with hereditary depression. She sees several psychiatrists, spends time in several asylums, and finally drowns in what is reported to be a scuba diving accident. After two years of imagining that her depression and death were his fault, Albert finally finds out from Christie that it had not been an accident but a carefully planned suicide. That knowledge seems to free him to fall in love with Lena.

There is more to the novel than that broad-stroke outline, but for purposes of this review, I need not say more than that. *The Diver* is only tangentially concerned with Parkinson's disease. The word Parkinson's itself is never used in the novel, but readers familiar with the disease will recognize the signs, right from the start:

> The old man walked through the garden with Ann. Her voice came to him from far away, as it often did. "Did you take your pills on schedule?" His steps were quite hesitant today, his progress labored. He wobbled from one side to the other, stopped, then hurried on after her. (5)

> He stumbled, quickly thrust his cane forward while his left hand clutched her for support. [...] "Did you take your pills?" she persisted. (7)

> Were his hands trembling again? Was that starting up again? He put them under the table, resting them on his knees. Don't get up now, he thought, that will just make it worse. (9)

> That evening he was in the bathroom trying to unbutton his shirt, but his fingers had lost their strength and were fluttering wildly again. He sat down heavily on the chair that had been shoehorned into the cramped space just for him. His pants had fallen to the floor and were bunched around his ankles. He bent down to free his feet, tugging impatiently at the pant legs until they finally gave in and he was holding the wrinkled pants in his hand trying to decide what to do with them. Should he get up, go into the dressing room, and hang them on the valet stand, or was it simpler to just drop them and undo the shirt buttons that were so uncooperative today? He heard her steps.
> "But, darling, why didn't you call me? How was I to know you were getting ready for bed so early today? How many times have I told you I'm happy to help? You need me!"
> He could hear the reproach in her voice. Ann stood next to him and had the shirt unbuttoned in a flash.
> "I wanted to do it myself. I just needed more time."
> "Admit that you can't do it alone anymore. It takes you forever!"

"It depends on the day. I don't usually need any help. I can handle things by myself."

"Why be so stubborn? Is it so hard to let someone help you? Don't be so pigheaded."

"What would you know about it?" he croaked, scratching his head.

She handed him his pajamas, picked up the pants, took his arm and walked him into the bedroom. (10–11)

No question about it—Albert has Parkinson's. But little is made of the fact that Albert has the disease. It does not appear to have directly influenced much of anything in the novel. It seems not, for example, to have influenced Albert's decision to give Lena up and return to the oppressive Ann. If he made that decision in part because Ann was better equipped to take care of an old man with Parkinson's, he never even comes close to acknowledging that fact.

C15. *A Misted Mirror*, by Gillian Jones. Hong Kong: Proverse Hong Kong, 2011. 169 pp.

"This ... disease; if that's what you call it. It's the wrong name, to me. A disease is something you can see, something like, well like the plague. That was a disease: boils and discoloured skin and scabs and things. But this; it's just a kind of crumbling away; an un-learning of everything he was good at."

Keith Jones was a little-known British poet. As a young man he had lived for a time in Nigeria, teaching and doing linguistics and language acquisition research. Then he worked in London, then in Tehran, then back in London. His marriage to a first wife did not last, but in Tehran he met Gillian, the woman who would become his second wife, the mother of their two sons, his caregiver after he was diagnosed with Parkinson's in his early fifties, his widow, his sort-of biographer, and his poetry anthologizer. The title of Gillian Jones's book is a paraphrase of a line from "Koi," one of the many poems by her husband that she publishes in her book: "life is this / misted mirror" (9).

A Misted Mirror might best be described as a fictionalized memoir. For reasons of her own, Gillian Jones is reluctant to narrate the memoir in her own voice, and so adopts the name "Sarah." She explains it this way in her prologue:

> With a deep distrust of memory and awareness of the pitfalls awaiting the first-person narrator, I personally am deterred from the attempt to tell this story and I have decided instead to hand the task over to "Sarah." "David" becomes the subject of the story and Sarah, the wife, is the one to tell it. Maybe we can take the facts on trust from Sarah as she recalls them, with a minimum of hesitation or self-interrogation. If the reader wants to question anyone about anything at all, let him or her question Sarah. (11)

Sarah tells us that David is "the subject of the story," but that is not really true. David's story remains pretty misted throughout. We ultimately do learn through Sarah a good bit about him, but more memorable is what we learn about Sarah herself, who becomes the real subject of the story. When, for example, David's Parkinson's makes him freeze, we learn more about Sarah's frustration with Parkinson's than about David's:

> The times, for example when his apparent immobility appeared to be more willful bloody-mindedness and a determination not to be helpful than the effects of his disease, those times when he stood stock-still, like a statue and transfixed, when only a moment ago hadn't he been hopping around the kitchen? Or in the bedroom, trying to get him dressed in the morning and he suddenly refused to move. Those were the moments when my temper snapped and, "Oh for Christ's sake David, why can't you bloody well put your own socks on!" escaped me as a moment of blessed relief. (13)

We learn less about what Parkinson's does to David than about what it does to his wife. Sarah later tells their friend Colin, "at one moment I'm so sorry for him and the next he's driving me mad!" (37). The sorry is muted; the mad is loud and clear.

To say that this book is less David's story than is Sarah's is not to criticize *A Misted Mirror* or its author. One of the nastiest tragedies of Parkinson's disease is that it devastates not only or even primarily the one with the tremors. It also devastates the people who are responsible for seeing to the care of the person who has the tremors—and the stumbling and the freezing and the stiffness and the falling and the hallucinations and the dementia—not to mention the worry and the despair and the expense of it all. Sarah is to be commended for being honest about her own frustrations as primary caregiver.

When she decides that taking care of David at home is too much for her, she makes arrangements for him to be cared for in a nearby nursing home. She at first feels desperate, guilty, fractured. She reports that one of the receiving nurses had told her: "Do you know, when you came in here first, you looked as if you were ready either to cut his throat or your own!" (14). A few months later, the staff of the nursing home finds reason to refuse to take care of David any longer and sends him home. We can only guess how David felt about that move, if he was even aware of it. But we find out loud and clear how Sarah felt: "When David came back from the nursing home that first time I was in a panic: resentful, bitter, feeling trapped—everything" (66). She goes on to talk about her feelings of "self-pity, guilt, grief, and all the many emotions that had been building up" (67).

When David finally dies—of pneumonia, it turns out—it is difficult not to feel a sense of relief to realize that David's journey is over, but also that Sarah will now have a chance to chart a journey of her own. It is not surprising that part of that journey involves writing this book about David. To tell it Sarah searches her memory, examines David's medical records, reads his poems, visits places he once lived, and consults some of his old friends to try to find out what her husband's early life had been like before she met him in Tehran. From those misty materials she fashions some of the facts of his life. What she finds out about him is interesting enough, and it helps us to make some sense of David's—that is, Keith Jones's—often-obscure poems that she reproduces at the start of each chapter. But it also helps us to understand what her own life as a caregiver is like.

A Misted Mirror also gives us a fresh window on what Parkinson's disease is like and the devastation it wreaks. When David's old friend Colin visits David and Sarah, he questions Sarah about David's Parkinson's disease: "This ... disease; if that's what you call it. It's the wrong name, to me. A disease is something you can see, something like, well like the plague. That was a disease: boils and discoloured skin and scabs and things. But this; it's just a kind of crumbling away; an un-learning of everything he was good at" (36). Not a bad way to describe Parkinson's: a process of un-learning, an education-in-reverse, growing up backwards, a growing down.

C16. *The Quality of Light*, by Richard Collins. Bridgend, Wales: Poetry Wales Press, 1911. 196 pp.

"He is thinking about suicide. It is not an urgent thought; he is not ready to die just yet. But it is an idea for the future, for the time when he is unable to do anything at all and there is no point in living."

Six years before the present-time action of *The Quality of Light*, an artist-teacher named Michael Marantz had directed a week-long creative-experience seminar for a group of arts-oriented young people. Among them were a young man named Daniel Brownlow and a young woman named Isabel Davies. Now Daniel drifts back to the Welsh seaport city where the course had been set. He comes ostensibly to house-sit for a friend of a friend for a week, but really to rethink his life. Meanwhile, Isabel decides to return to the same city to buy a house and start a new life. Daniel and Isabel are both still trying to figure out who they are, what they want to do with their lives, and who they want to do it with. Daniel has meanwhile drifted into an ambiguous relationship with a woman named Sarah who has a two-year-old daughter, and Isabel has drifted into an ambiguous relationship with a man named Max. The major tension in this novel of self-rediscovery is the developing romance between Daniel and Isabel. Will they figure out a way, after not seeing each other for six years, to take advantage of a second week together to consummate a friendship that has lain dormant?

More interesting is their former teacher. Michael is now "a sturdy middle-aged man with a broad face, salt-and-pepper stubble on his chin, thick grey hair. [...] He walks with a limp; his right leg drags a little. He is somewhat lopsided and unsteady" (15). The problem is that "he has recently been diagnosed with a seriously bad-shit degenerative disease and his outlook is bleak" (16). Michael is by profession a painter, but his Parkinson's interferes with his ability to paint: "The stiffness and pain in his hands have increased. He can paint but it hurts. And he knows this will get worse and then go on getting worse. He will not be able to do the few things that he is able to do now" (37).

Michael has lived alone for some time, ever since his infidelity has brought about a separation from his wife Christina. He misses their daughter Zoë. He still occasionally gets together with his ex-wife. In one such meeting Christina asks Michael about his health. He replies:

"It's downhill but it's a very slow downhill. I'm all right and I'll go on being all right for quite awhile, I hope." As he speaks he is aware that this is not the whole truth. There are days when he feels things are getting worse more quickly than he'd anticipated. It feels better not to say that. (59)

What bothers Michael most about his Parkinson's is the little things, like his failed attempt at the post office to mail a package to his daughter:

He pushes forward a ten-pound note that he had taken out of his wallet well in advance. The woman passes the stamps and his change through to him. And it all feels like it's too much. He has to collect the coins together and put them in his pocket and his left hand isn't really working at all. He drops a pound coin on the floor and manages to pick it up again. But now he must stick the stamps on before handing over the parcel and he knows he can't do it. He feels confused, snatches at the stamps, crumples them up in his hand and walks out hurriedly, still carrying the parcel. […] What hurts the most is the fact that he is losing the ability to give, to do something for others. He wanted to send a present to someone he loves and he couldn't do it. He feels that he has let Zoë down again. (83)

Not surprisingly, Michael contemplates the means to an early exit. One day he makes his way to the edge of a high cliff and sits on a rock:

He is thinking about suicide. It is not an urgent thought; he is not ready to die just yet. But it is an idea for the future, for the time when he is unable to do anything at all and there is no point in living. Except that if he is unable to do anything then he won't be able to get himself here to bring things to an end. Unless they have installed wheelchair access by then to allow the disabled the same choices as everyone else. Equal opportunities, that's right, isn't it? Michael laughs out loud. (102)

A little humor—even dark humor—is a healthy sign. Michael's ability to find something to laugh about as he contemplates suicide is a positive development.

By the end there are hints that Michael may eventually be reconciled with his ex-wife if only so that they can together help their daughter Zoë through a difficult time in her own life. In the last chapter, Christina tells Michael that she has told Zoë that her parents both love her and that Michael's Parkinson's "isn't as bad as it sounds and that you would be OK for a long time. Decades, perhaps." Michael replies, "I think that might be true. I've heard that it can be very slow. But I've been funny about it. I've been doing the head-in-the–sand-thing, trying not to think about it but meanwhile imagining it's worse than it really is" (193). That is not a super-cheerful ending, but it is something. We can imagine, if we want to, that Michael will not be entirely alone in the difficult times—decades, perhaps—that lie ahead for him.

C17 *Take the Lead*, by Johnny Diaz. Frisco, Texas: Dreamspinner Press, 2011. 225 pp.

> "I love my father with all my heart, and if I could yank that horrible disease out of his body, I would. I'd fight it and win. But it's Papi who is quietly engaged in his own private battle with his body."

If you wanted to write a novel about the love life of a handsome, lonely, gay, single middle-aged professor who teaches journalism and creative writing at a college in Boston, but you wanted your novel to convey a lot of information about Parkinson's disease, what kind of novel would you write? Answer: you would write a novel like *Take the Lead*. The narrator and main character of Johnny Diaz's novel is a thirty-five-year-old Cuban-American professor named Gabriel Galan. Gabriel is troubled by the fact that, while he has had a number of sexual partners, he has not found his Mr. Right. When one of his former students, a handsome twenty-two-year-old named Craig begins flirting with him, Gabriel welcomes his advances. He knows that Craig is too young for him and he knows that it is ethically questionable for a teacher to date a former student, but he cannot resist the handsome Craig. Gabriel worries that his hair is starting to get grey and takes medicines to head off baldness. He is flattered to realize that Craig finds him attractive, and eagerly responds to his overtures.

Gabriel's aunt calls him from Florida to tell him that his father's Parkinson's seems to be getting worse. Gabriel decides to fly home at Thanksgiving to Fort Lauderdale to visit his parents, who are divorced. He gives us a bit of his family history:

> My father, Guillermo Galan, is a hard-working exterminator despite
> having Parkinson's disease, which he's been able to keep at bay
> over the years. The disease's assault on his body has been a slow but
> persistent march, from what I can tell. My mother, Gladys, is strong
> and healthy, too. […] I adore my parents even though at times I feel
> like I'm in a perpetual tug of war between them. That's one of the
> reasons I chose to move away and be on my own in New England.
> (5)

Not surprisingly, we find out that Guillermo's lifetime of exterminating
cockroaches in Florida is almost certainly what caused his Parkinson's. We
do not find out until later that the reason Gabriel's parents have divorced
is that Guillermo had had an apparently short-lived affair with another
woman. Gabriel wishes he could do more for his dad than visit him a couple
of times a year:

> I love my father with all my heart, and if I could yank that horrible
> disease out of his body, I would. I'd fight it and win. But it's Papi
> who is quietly engaged in his own private battle with his body. I
> would use every bit of my strength to help him. (31)

Gabriel eventually tells Craig why he is heading for Florida. It turns out that
Craig is sympathetic because his grandmother had Parkinson's:

> Craig places a comforting hand on my right shoulder. "My
> grandmother had Parkinson's too. I know what my mom, aunts, and
> uncles had to deal with, so you have my sympathy. […] She was
> in a wheelchair and had trouble breathing. It's a horrible disease.
> I watched her lose control of her body. No one should have to go
> through that." (49–50)

I use the verb "shoe-horn" to describe a fiction-writer's effort to squeeze
factual information into a story. To give himself a chance to shoe-horn
into his novel some more information about the disease, Johnny Diaz has
Gabriel go to his college library to do some research:

> I spent an hour Googling different organizations, support groups,
> and various definitions of the disease. I learned that despite all the
> research, there's still no cure for Parkinson's, which affects more
> than 1.5 million Americans. Like Papi, most patients take a daily

mix of pills that slow the progress of the disease, which occurs when brain cells that produce dopamine die off. Dopamine is a naturally produced chemical that transmits the signals that control muscle movement. When dopamine-producing cells are destroyed, people start to lose their balance, coordination, and muscle control. (54)

Another instance of shoe-horning comes when Gabriel, in Florida visiting his father, takes him for a consultation with his neurologist, who talks about the importance of exercise: "Are you exercising, Guillermo? Nice long walks at night and riding a bicycle, even stationary one, will loosen some of your stiffness" (88).

Perhaps the most egregious instance of shoe-horning comes when Gabriel is back in Boston. He invites Tommy Perez, a practicing journalist, to talk to his class. At the end of Tommy's lecture, one of the students asks Tommy what stories he is working on now:

> "Well, I'm writing a story about a special dance class for people with Parkinson's. It takes place in Cambridge. The class is designed to help Parkinsonians relax and loosen their muscles, but the dancing also lifts their spirits. You see, a lot of Parkinson's patients tend to isolate themselves and suffer from depression because of their condition." (98)

Gabriel, who has never heard of that class, decides to visit it. By now he has discovered that the handsome young Craig has been flirting with and dating other men. Gabriel is excited by the class and its teacher, "a yoga and dance instructor named Adam Smith who incorporates movements from each of those disciplines to help people with Parkinson's improve their coordination and flexibility as the disease gradually robs them of both" (117). Gabriel is drawn to Adam, an age-appropriate gay man who likes him also. In the end, Gabriel arranges for both his father and his mother to fly up to Boston to visit the class and meet his lover Adam. Apparently we are to imagine that Guillermo will be helped by the dancing, that he and Gladys will be reconciled, that she will return to Florida with him to be his caregiver, and that Gabriel and Adam will thus be free to live happily ever after in Boston.

C18. *The Wreckage,* by Michael Robotham. New York: Mulholland Books (Little, Brown), 2011. 439 pp.

> "He shakes it like Shakira when he's not medicated."

Joe O'Loughlin appears on only a half-dozen pages of *The Wreckage*. He has almost nothing to do with the various plot lines of this international thriller. We are told in the first of his brief appearances that he is "a clinical psychologist who spends too much time in other people's heads. He looks exactly like you'd expect an academic to look—disheveled, unkempt, undernourished—only he has Parkinson's which means he shakes it like Shakira when he's not medicated" (115). Vincent Ruiz, one of the focal characters, is said to have "met him eight years ago, when he was investigating the murder of a young woman in London"—a reference to the events in *Suspect*. That would make Joe around fifty in this novel.

C19. *Dutch Island,* by Curt Weeden. Mount Pleasant, South Carolina: Quadrafoil Press, 2012. xi + 246 pp.

> "Doc would later explain that an involuntary closure of the eyes was called blepharospasm and it was just one of the miserable maladies brought on by Parkinson's disease."

On a dark night when Richard Bullock, the vacationing manager of a New Jersey men's shelter, is surf-fishing on a beach in Narragansett Bay, a stranger gives him some uninvited advice about how to fish. A few minutes later the stranger is murdered—indeed almost beheaded—by someone wielding a hatchet. A neighbor named Roger Standish calls the police and reports that the victim is a corrupt local real estate developer named Harold Mason, who is in partnership with his two sons, Caleb Mason and J. D. Mason. The Masons are trying to negotiate the sale of Dutch Island, a small island in the bay, to an Arab multi-billionaire named Mohammed al-Tabal, who wants to build a lavish mosque there and construct a three-mile undersea tunnel out to it. Other characters include a titty-bar mob-boss named Manny Maglio, his niece, a bleach blonde, size-D-boobed ex-stripper and prostitute named Twyla Tharp, recently impregnated by her Jewish husband, a lawyer named Yigal Rosenblatt. Then there is Doug Kool, Bullock's friend, who has arranged for Bullock to house-sit for two weeks at the Rhode Island waterside mansion of two other friends of his, Kenneth and Maureen O'Connor, while they travel in Europe. Part of the house-sitting deal is that Bullock is to take care of Olive, the O'Connor's poodle. We also have Alyana Genesee, the next-door veterinarian neighbor, descended from Pequot and Narragansett Indians. She looks after Olive when Bullock is being interrogated by the local police lieutenant, a black man named Michael Ravenel, who assumes that Bullock is the murderer of Harold Mason.

Confused? That is just the first two chapters—thirteen pages. There are more characters and more deaths to come as the story-line develops: the old Narragansett Indian Lloyd Noka, who is soon found hanging dead in his home—apparently a suicide but really a murder; William Nonesuch, who claims to be a Narragansett but is not; Charles Kenyon, a belligerent drunk who drives his pickup truck into a big oak tree—"the side of the man's head was crushed, one eye and half his jaw pulverized" (55); Doc "One-Nut" Waters, an ex-Rutgers history professor whose gambling addiction had led his enemies to punish him by using a pair of pliers to squeeze one of his gonads "until it burst with sickening pop and sent such an agonizing bolt of pain through the spermatic plexus that Doc went unconscious" (79). Bullock enlists Doc Waters's help in locating an early deed to Dutch Island, a deed that might prevent its sale to the Arab. Later still we meet Aurelie and Yves Benoit when Bullock and Alyana go to their restaurant for a delicious meal. While they are enjoying their dinner someone drives a car over the head of J. D. Mason, the younger son of Harold Mason, and then smears some of his brain matter on the front fender of Bullock's parked car so it will look as if he were the killer.

Following all that we continue to meet new characters: Tommy Caddefield and Frank Purvis, who apparently killed Lloyd Noka; Miriam Constable Reis, the librarian who locates the missing deed; Destiny, who holds a baby shower for Twyla, her former call-girl colleague; Saul Lipschitz, who has a pet female ferret named Ellie Weasel; Tiny Templeton, a three-hundred-pound man who, when Ellie Weasel runs up his pant-leg, tries to shoot the ferret but shoots himself by mistake and bleeds to death.

About now you are probably wondering two things. First, is *Dutch Island* some kind of a farce? And, second, does *Dutch Island* have any connection with Parkinson's disease? The answer to the first question is,

Yes. The answer to the second question is, Not yet.

The answer to both questions can be found in the first three sentences of Curt Weedon's "Author's Epilogue": "To the publishing trade, *Dutch Island* is a comedic mystery. But this novel has deeper roots. Woven through the fiction are historical facts, including medical truths, and a real-life tale of profound love and courage" (233). The historical part he goes on in the epilogue to outline: the history of the actual Dutch Island in Narragansett Bay and his own family's role in that history, starting in 1657, when a Quaker named William Weeden became part owner of the island. The "medical truths" and the "real-life tale of profound love and courage" do not enter the novel until the final six chapters.

None of the many, many characters I have been describing in the first twenty chapters (the first 167 pages), mentions even one word about Parkinson's disease. In Chapter 21, however, we meet two new characters, Betty Weeden and Rick Weeden: "Alyana had told me about the man's advanced Parkinson's disease. The Weedens had been married for nearly forty-five years and for all that time but fifteen, Rick had battled a debilitating sickness that tore at his central nervous system" (169). The narrator Bullock serves up a few more medical facts: "Rick's face briefly showed the same apprehension and then his eyelids clamped shut. Doc would later explain that an involuntary closure of the eyes was called blepharospasm and it was just one of the miserable maladies brought on by Parkinson's disease" (171). Later, when Rick Weedon's leg jerks out, Bullock tells us, "It was a spastic, involuntary movement called dyskinesia common to many Parkinson's patients" (174). Later still, Betty explains some of the difficulties her husband faced:

> On the drive to the campground, Betty had explained that like many Parkinson's patients, Rick had trouble speaking. "Getting the words out is hardly the worst of it," she had said and explained how tremors, stiff muscles, and drooling made Rick's life a living hell. "But it's the hallucinations, depression, and anxiety that turn everything into a nightmare."
>
> "I can't imagine what that must be like," I had reacted. "With everything else he's dealing with, Rick still manages a smile. He's pretty amazing." As is his wife, I thought. (179)

It is a bit of a stretch, but author Curt Weedon finds a way to let his two real-life relatives help solve the fictional comedic mystery and even play a role in bringing the main killer to justice. I have no desire to divulge too much of the ending, but Betty skippers the little boat that carries a brave coterie of characters across stormy waters to Dutch Island. And then, on the island, Rick cleverly figures out a way to get Ellie Weasel, the pet ferret, to disarm the murderous bad guy so that he—Rick—can use his broken cane to rip open his—the bad guy's—guts.

In the "Author's Note" at the beginning of the novel Curt Weeden reports that, "Rick Weeden who inspired this novel lost his battle with Parkinson's disease on March 13, 2013. [...] Like the fictional character of this book, Rick showed courage and resolve that truly made him a hero" (v).

It seems that Curt Weeden had too many goals in *Dutch Island*: to tell a spoof-murder mystery; to describe the history of a real island; to work in some facts about Parkinson's disease; and to honor two of his own admired relatives. In trying to accomplish too much, he accomplished too little.

C20. *Love is Two People Talking,* by Charles H. Banov, MD. Charleston, South Carolina: Evening Post Books, 2012. 115 pp.

> "You have to do your part—which includes maintaining a positive attitude. Remember, if you give up, you lose."
>
> "And if I don't, I'll win?"
>
> "If you don't give up, you'll come back to see me again."

I tend to be suspicious of a novel that announces its major theme in its title. I mean, why bother to read the whole book if you know right off that true love is based on communication or, conversely, that if you cannot talk to a person you can scarcely be said to love him or her?

The focal character in the novel is its narrator, an eighty-year-old Jewish pawnbroker named Sam Geller. The important people in his life are his wife, Sandy, who died seven years earlier, their son Jeffrey, a dermatologist, Jeffrey's wife Carol, their two daughters Kate and Peggy, and Sam Geller's newly-found girlfriend, an age-appropriate widow named Irene Kurtz. Of these, the three people that Sam most needs to learn to love-talk with are Irene, Jeffrey, and Peggy.

Sam succeeds pretty well in his love-talking with Irene. He takes her out, has long chats with her, has dinner at her house, and sleeps over. He gets lots of positive reinforcement from her, as when she tells him, "You're a good man, Sam Geller, You're a very good man" (75).

Sam does not succeed all that well with his son Jeffrey. They try to talk, but have little to say to one another and generally feel awkward in each other's company.

As for talking with his granddaughter Peggy, no one succeeds in talking with her because she is incapable of speech. Peggy suffers from a nasty disease called Rett syndrome, a medical condition akin to autism: "Peggy couldn't speak; her spine was bent; she could hardly walk. Her feet were splayed and she dragged one of them. She always hung her head like she was ashamed. She had difficulty swallowing" (58). Peggy can perhaps understand some things that others try to say to her, but she is incapable of speech herself—unless we count screaming as a form of speech. When anyone comes near her, touches her, or even looks her in the eye, Peggy screams. Sam forms a kind of distant friendship with Peggy, and he sometimes thinks that he can read the "language" conveyed in her looks, scowls, and screams. That is not really two people talking, but the author invites us to expand the meaning of "talking" so that it includes telepathy. Sam's doctor puts it this way when he speaks to Sam about his closeness to Peggy: "Since you've been diagnosed with Parkinson's a kind of telepathy has developed between the two of you" (96). If one person trying to interpret the pre-lingual gesticulating of another counts as talking, then Sam's strange friendship with his granddaughter counts as love-talk.

There is no cure for Rett syndrome. Most people who have it die before they are ten. Peggy is already twenty-five, yet still she cannot talk, dress herself, or change her own diapers. The most important moral dilemma in the novel is whether the family should put Peggy in a nearby care facility. They carefully weigh Peggy's needs against the needs of the rest of the family. They hesitate, waver, feel guilty, then finally decide to put her in the care facility. Then—well never mind. Read *Love Is Two People Talking* for yourself if you want to know what happens to Peggy.

If you do read it, you will discover that the novel showcases two kinds of illness, Rett syndrome and Parkinson's disease. That is not surprising in view of the fact that Charles Banov, the author of this, his first, novel is a retired medical doctor. That his description of Rett syndrome is so detailed and convincing is explained by the fact that one of Dr. Banov's own six children had Rett syndrome.

Dr. Banov's discussion of Parkinson's disease is less convincing. Much of his information seems to come out of a medical textbook:

> I freeze suddenly in mid-stride as if my shoes were covered with glue and stuck to the pavement. It takes me twice as long now to get out of bed in the morning and dress myself. I'm unsteady on my feet. Sometimes I suddenly lose my balance and fall. I'm forgetful and have difficulty swallowing. My handwriting looks like a doctor's prescription. (6)

> It wasn't long afterward that my own health began to fail, slowly at first, but steadily. Parkinson's is destroying my motor skills primarily, abilities I once took for granted—like walking with ease, talking without a struggle, and standing tall and steady. This disease has stolen almost everything from me. (8)

> I've accepted the fact that I have Parkinson's disease and it will not go away—that it affects my brain and my signals get crossed at times; that my muscles are shutting down; that I drool occasionally and have difficulty swallowing. The tremors will continue. [...] I'm slowly losing my senses. I never know what to expect, I'm too hot one day, too cold the next. I always carry a sweater with me now, even in August when the thermometer hits 100 degrees. My vision is blurred sometimes. (76-77)

To be sure, those are all legitimate symptoms of Parkinson's. There are, however, two problems. One is that Sam Geller, who is not diagnosed until he is eighty, unrealistically presents all those symptoms right away, not gradually over a period of years. Another problem is that Sam is still driving his car. Why is an eighty-year-old man with all those symptoms—tremors, freezing, blurred vision, shut-down muscles, crossed brain signals, glued-down feet, not to mention a broken wrist —-doing behind the wheel?

Near the end of the novel Sam, having noticed that his symptoms are getting worse, goes to see his neurologist. The doctor confirms that his symptoms are indeed getting worse, but he tells Sam not to give up in his apparently hopeless struggle with Parkinson's:

> "You have to do your part—which includes maintaining a positive attitude. Remember, if you give up, you lose."
> "And if I don't, I'll win?"
> "If you don't give up, you'll come back to see me again." (95)

That is the reward? Wow.

C21. *Say You're Sorry*, by Michael Robotham. New York: Mulholland Books (Little, Brown), 2012. 439 pp.

> "One day, not so many years from now, you'll be a jerking, shitting, quivering sack of bones, unable to walk or talk or feed yourself."

In *Say You're Sorry* two fifteen-year-old girls, Natasha "Tash" McBain and Piper Hadley, disappear. Most people assume that they have run away and will return when they run out of money, but they do not come back—not for three years. It is gradually revealed that they had been drugged and abducted by a psychopath who squirrels them away for three years in a cold, dungeon-like basement in an abandoned nuclear research facility not far from their home. Neither Tash nor Piper knows who he is or what his name is. They assign him a nickname "George."

Their unheated basement home has a propane stove and two cot beds. Though it has a small high window, the room itself is accessible only by a trap door in the high ceiling, a door held closed by heavy furniture that George places above it. George comes and moves the furniture from time to time to open the trap door so he can check on the girls. He brings them food (mostly canned beans) and magazines. On some of these visits he drops a rope down so he can lift out the rancid contents of their chamber pot. Sometimes he calls Tash, the prettier of the two girls, to join him upstairs. He lets her take a warm bath, gives her a decent meal, and rapes her. Then he sends her back down again. This bizarre behavior goes on for three years. Finally, after he performs a clitorectomy on her, the distraught Tash manages to slither out the window and escape, but George finds her and chases her to a frozen pond where she drowns.

The police find the frozen body and eventually identify the dead woman as Tash McBain. That raises the question of where Piper Hadley is. Is she dead? Is she alive somewhere? Had she perhaps not run away from home after all, but been abducted by the same person who had murdered Tash? Does George rape her as he had raped Tash? We readers know the answers to some of these questions because we get to read alternating italicized chapters in which Piper tells her story, but Joe O'Loughlin, Vincent Ruiz, and the local police have to figure it all out. They do, of course, but you won't hear the details from me. Nope. No way. I will say only that the plot is unlikely (why does it take three years for Tash to figure out how to wriggle out the little window?); the motivation of George is opaque (why

does he carry out his three-year reign of terror against these two women?);
Joe seems unusually plodding (why, once he finds Piper, does he leave her
alone to be seized again by George?); and Julianne's motivation seems ever
more opaque (why, after spurning him for three years, does she invite Joe
back into her bed again in the final scene?).

But this review is mostly about another question: how important is
Joe's Parkinson's in *Say You're Sorry*? The answer is, not very. We find
occasional references to arm tremors (182, 297), to pill rolling (53), to "on"
and "off" periods (22, 277, 388), to the Parkinson's "mask" (70), and to
difficulties buttoning shirts (198). Joe tells someone that he was diagnosed
eight years earlier but is still in "stage one" (182). For the first time, Joe
mentions his specific medications and his problems with depression:
"Levodopa for the symptoms, carbidopa for the nausea, Prozac to stop me
being depressed about having a major degenerative illness" (54). The most
interesting reference to Joe's Parkinson's comes near the end when Joe has
a conversation with a research scientist named Phillip Martinez. Thinking
that Martinez may be the "George" who had abducted Tash and Piper, Joe
purposefully angers the scientist, eliciting a furiously unfiltered response:

> "How dare you insult me and question my ethics. Look at you!
> You're diseased! You're only functioning because of the drugs
> that people like me have discovered and tested. Your condition is
> getting worse—eating away at your nerves, robbing you of balance,
> movement, speech and eventually your mind. One day, not so many
> years from now, you'll be a jerking, shitting, quivering sack of
> bones, unable to walk or talk or feed yourself. Instead of insulting
> my reputation, you should be praying I find a cure. You should
> be begging for my help, you pompous, self-righteous schmuck."
> (395–96).

Joe's response is intellectual, a professional analysis of the limitations of
the speaker: "I recognize a classic narcissist, a perfectionist governed by
his own ego and sense of worth, someone who cannot accept anyone who
questions the carefully crafted, flawless image he has manufactured of
himself. He will destroy the messenger, rather than hear the message" (396).

Joe never seems to realize that that is precisely what he himself is doing.
Instead of responding to the message Martinez is giving him about what
lies ahead for people with Parkinson's, Joe attacks the character of the
messenger. Readers who would want to know Joe's emotional and personal

reaction to the content of Martinez's prediction about what Joe's end—and theirs—may be like will be disappointed.

C22. *Watching You*, by Michael Robotham. New York: Mulholland Books (Little, Brown), 2013. 421 pp.

> "How would he shoulder a burden like Joe's? Would he cope as all sufferers cope—because he had no choice—or would he crawl into a hole and never come out?"

The beautiful Marnella "Marnie" Logan is a psychological mess. Ever since her husband, Daniel Hyland, disappeared a year earlier, she has been receiving counseling twice a week by clinical psychologist Joe O'Loughlin, Joe is beginning to think that Marnie has multiple personalities.

A compulsive gambler, Daniel Hyland had lost all of their savings and had then disappeared, leaving his wife Marnie with no money, no job, heavy debts, and two children to raise—a fifteen-year-old daughter named Zoe and a four-year-old son named Elijah. Because of her husband's gambling debts—for example, she owes a man named Patrick Hennessy upwards of thirty thousand pounds—Marnie decides to become a prostitute in order to pay the bills. One of her first clients is a depressed middle-aged man named Owen. Owen's mother has recently died. Marnie soon discovers that Owen is so upset that he plans to commit suicide by jumping into the Thames. She talks him out of that plan. He decides not to have sex with her but wants to pay her anyhow. Marnie refuses to accept the money. For her generosity, she is later beaten up by Niall Quinn, her pimp. Not long after that, Niall Quinn is found floating in the Thames, his throat cut.

Trevor Waite, the maintenance man in the apartment building where Marnie and her children live, makes an aggressive pass at Marnie. She fights him off and leaves him writhing in pain. The next day he is found dead in his apartment, both his hands cut off. Patrick Hennessy tries to collect sexual favors from Marnie as partial repayment for some of the thirty thousand pounds that he says Marnie owes him. He also turns up dead—his head twisted almost off.

Joe O'Loughlin and Vincent Ruiz become involved with the local police officers in trying to figure why all these men are being murdered.

The police, led by Detective Inspector Gennia, quickly conclude that Marnie herself committed the murders and also must also have murdered her husband Daniel: "That woman is a cold-blooded killer" (303), Gennia declares. Joe and Vincent, are not so sure.

It is not surprising that Joe and Vincent turn out to be right and that Marnie is innocent of those murders. What is surprising is that Owen, the man who was depressed by his aging mother's death and planned to drown himself after he had purchased the sexual favors of a prostitute named Marnie, turns out to be Marnie's father and thus the grandfather of Zoe and Elijah. Who would have guessed?

I could tell you who murdered all those men and abducts Owen's daughters and grandchildren, and carries them off to an isolated cabin in the woods, but you wouldn't believe me. You would also not believe me if I told you who cuts out Owen's eyeballs with shards of a broken mirror.

Joe still misses Julianne, but she refuses to let him move back in with her and his daughters. He explains to Ruiz that "We're not sleeping together." "Not even accidentally bumping into each other in the dark?" Ruiz asks. "Afraid not," Joe answers (114).

Joe still has Parkinson's in *Watching You*, but it does not much influence the action or outcome of the novel. He still refers to his disease as "Mr. Parkinson" (53, 77, 163, 261). His left arm still has spasms (77), his shoulders still hunch forward (190), his face is still often mask-like (261), and he still freezes, stumbles and falls (33, 163). Joe continues to get some relief from his medications, when he remembers to take them:

> Joe's left arm is jerking spasmodically, his medication wearing off. He should have taken a pill earlier. Feeling in his pocket, he searches for the small white plastic bottle. Managing to get it open, he swallows the pill dry, waiting for the chemicals in his brain to rebalance. (184)

Joe sometimes has trouble speaking, making him sound retarded to some local drunkards who harass him about his strange behavior:

> Joe's right hand opens unconsciously and his white pill bottle bounces across the asphalt and rolls toward a grated drain. One of them places his heel on the bottle. Joe's tongue has grown fat and lazy in his mouth making his words thick and wet. "Please don't do that."
>
> "You a retard?" asks one of them.

"No."

"I hate retards." [. . .]

The boot presses down, crushing the bottle and grinding the contents into a powdery dust that seems to glow in the darkness. (185)

Joe seems to be more aware of his medications in this novel, and of the side-effects of those medications, one of which is drooling: "A bubble of spit forms on his lips because his medication produces excess saliva" (396).

I sense that Michael Robotham is not sure quite what to do with Joe's Parkinson's in this novel. I sense that he would like to be able to leave it behind since it has very little bearing on much of anything in these novels, but he cannot do that. Joe has the disease and there is no cure, so Joe, like the rest of us, has to keep on having it. If a cure were available, Joe could be rid of Mr. Parkinson. But it is not: "He knows that science moves slower than the disease" (77). Robotham does have Ruiz wonder how he would respond to the diagnosis that Joe received eight years earlier: "How would he shoulder a burden like Joe's? Would he cope as all sufferers cope—because he had no choice—or would he crawl into a hole and never come out?" (190).

C23. *Close Your Eyes*, by Michael Robotham. New York: Mulholland Books (Little, Brown), 2015. 383 pp.

> "Existence has become infinitely more complex
> and less joyful. Mr. Parkinson has become my
> cellmate and we're serving 'life' together."

What sort of man would use a box-cutter knife to carve the letter "A" into the foreheads of his victims, then let them go? What sort of man would murder the forty-four-year-old Elizabeth Crowe by stabbing her thirty-six times with a seven-inch-long kitchen knife, then decorate the crime scene with candles? What sort of man would choke Elizabeth's seventeen-year-old daughter Harper Crowe and then leave her body beautifully laid out as if she were a sleeping princess? Those are some of the questions that face Joe O'Loughlin in *Close Your Eyes*, the eighth novel in a series in which the psychologist teams up with his trusted friend Vincent Ruiz to solve a bizarre series of crimes that baffle the local police.

In this novel Robotham continues his technique of taking his readers into the twisted mind and contorted motives of the criminal by giving us a series of italicized chapters narrated by him. We learn, for example, that when the criminal was just a boy of seven his mother had been killed in an automobile accident while giving oral sex to the driver of the automobile, and that as she died she had bitten off his penis. We learn that the boy's father had been so angered and humiliated by that event that he took his frustration out in acts of cruelty to his children, belittling them and beating them. We learn that his father has eventually been diagnosed with dementia and sent to a nursing home. We learn that the now-grown-up son, in a twisted act of revenge against his promiscuous mother, had set out on a one-man campaign to sniff out and punish other adulterers.

We readers, then, know a lot about this criminal before Joe does. We know that he likes to waylay his victims along a certain isolated footpath. We know that he is especially harsh in punishing men and women who engage in "dogging"—that is, who like to have sexual intercourse in public places in full view of others. We know that he has perfected the technique of "blood-choking"—cutting off the flow of blood to the brain long enough for him to carve a scarlet "A" for "Adultery" in his victim's foreheads, before letting the blood flow back to their brains so they can recover consciousness after he has disappeared. We know that he sometimes keeps the blood-choke pressure on until his victims die. We know a lot about him, but not his name or who he is or how he is related—if he is—to Elizabeth and Harper Crowe. That we learn only when Joe O'Loughlin figures it out near the very end, after the psychopath has kidnaped Joe's eighteen-year old daughter Charlie and his ten-year-old daughter Emma.

Except for the italicized chapters, *Close Your Eyes* is narrated by Joe O'Loughlin. Joe still refers to his disease from time to time. He recalls his reaction to his diagnosis ten years earlier (12). He still refers to his disease as "Mr. Parkinson" (51, 319, 371). He speaks of his shaking left arm (19, 31, 47, 116, 170), of the Parkinson's mask (38), of freezing (71), and of taking pills (9, 78).

I get the feeling that Robotham is about to kill off his Parkinsonian hero. Joe finds himself thinking that he is close to being an old man:

> I am not the same person I was a decade ago. Existence has become infinitely more complex and less joyful. Mr. Parkinson has become my cellmate and we're serving "life" together. Middle age is taking hold. I'm thinner, more stooped. [...] Old age is no longer a foreign

country that I hope to visit one day. It's over the horizon but on the
itinerary. (52)

When Joe's wife Julianne is diagnosed with ovarian cancer, she and Joe
have a discussion about human mortality. Julianne tells Joe about a news
story she had recently read:

> "It was about a woman who tried to talk a suicidal boy down
> from a rooftop. He jumped and she reached out and grabbed him by
> the belt, just in time. They were dangling off the side of the building
> until bystanders pulled them up. Afterwards, a reporter asked her
> whether she feared for her life and she said, 'We're all going to die.
> Why be frightened of it?'"
> "I wonder if she was dying," I reply.
> "What do you mean?"
> "People who are diagnosed with a terminal illness tend to show
> less regard for their personal safety. They know they're living on
> borrowed time." (129–30)

Joe clearly feels that he himself is living on borrowed time, and
he hopes to die before Julianne does: "The one small mercy of having
Parkinson's was the knowledge that I was likely to go first" (151). Later Joe
has a dream about Mr. Parkinson:

> In my dream Mr. Parkinson is a bent, crippled, skulking figure,
> the Gollum of my nightmares, scuttling after me, pulling at my
> body, trying to make me play with him. His arms and legs jerk
> in symmetry and he turns his eyes upon me, cocking his head in
> curiosity. "It won't be long," he says, "you'll be here soon." (319)

"Gollum," of course, is the dark underworld figure of evil who appears in
many of the works of J. R. R. Tolkien.

It is always dangerous to make predictions about books not yet written,
but I hereby predict that in the next novel in the Joe O'Loughlin series, Joe
will die in some heroic way. His death will not, however, bring the end to
the series, because I also predict that the series will continue, but with a
different Joe. The new Joe will be his daughter Charlie. Why else would
Robotham have Charlie come along as Joe's driver in *Close Your Eyes*,
demonstrate her mettle when she and Emma are seized by the killer, and
boldly announce her career plans to her father. She tells him that she wants

to attend Oxford to study psychology, and after that she wants to "get a doctorate and then study forensic psychology." Joe tries to dissuade her: "Forensic psychology is brutal. It's about delving into the worst of human behavior: sociopaths, psychopaths, rapists, pedophiles, abused children, victims of violence" (216).

Sounds like an advertisement for the next novel, doesn't it?

CPSIA information can be obtained
at www.ICGtesting.com
Printed in the USA
FFHW020153060719
53461209-59116FF

9 781603 817462